A Primer on

HEART DISEASE

for Patients and Their Families

Straight Talk from a Cardiologist
About Heart Disease,
How it is Diagnosed and Treated

Joe R. Wise, M.D., F.A.C.C.

PEAK PUBLISHING COMPANY
Ouray, Colorado

First Edition
Printed in the United States of America

ISBN 1-890437-28-X
Library of Congress Catalog Number 00-102173
Cover and text design by Laurie Goralka Design

Peak Publishing Company
P.O. Box 710
Ouray, CO 81427

For my father, who showed me how to be a doctor

"It has taken me a long time to learn that what has happened to me is of more importance to my patients than what I have read."

— Oliver Wendall Holmes

Author's Note

The reader will find some repetition of material throughout this book. This was done intentionally. It is anticipated that, while the book may be read by some in its entirety, others will read only selected chapters in which they are most interested. Therefore, the subject covered in each chapter is discussed thoroughly.

TABLE OF CONTENTS

⌒

PREFACE

Patients are often confused by the science and mystery of medicine. This unnecessary confusion is compounded by fear and sometimes by doctors who are either unable, or unwilling to explain. Actually, most things in medicine are logical and straightforward, and not nearly as complicated as they sometimes seem.

Nowhere in medicine is good communication more important than in talking with patients who have, or are afraid they have, heart disease, a modern epidemic which now kills more people each year than all other causes of death combined.

My goal in writing this book is to present a balanced and reasonable overview of some of the more common medical conditions affecting the heart in terms that, during my thirty years of cardiology practice, patients have told me they understood.

The topics covered are those which I have been asked about most often and include how the normal heart works, what can go wrong, how it can be diagnosed and what can be done about it. The liberal use of simple, clear illustrations helps clarify the scientific concepts for those without a science background.

Throughout the book I have strived to balance the scientific presentation with reason and common sense. While I have tried to show the potential dangers of heart disease, I have tried also to emphasize the optimism that we can now share about the treatment of heart disease as a result of the remarkable progress and promise of medical science and technology.

INTRODUCTION
What are we talking about here, anyway?

~

Death from heart disease has reached epidemic proportions. In the United States, as in most other industrialized nations, heart disease is the leading cause of death, killing more people each year than all the other causes of death put together.

In 1995, a year when 538,455 people died of cancer, cardiovascular diseases killed 960,592. By comparison, 49,000 died in US traffic accidents and 43,115 Americans died of AIDS.

Once only a killer of men, cardiovascular disease is now also the leading killer of American women, accounting for the deaths of 505,440 women per year compared to 256,844 for all forms of cancer.

The cost of caring for people with heart disease is staggering. It has been estimated that the medical costs due to heart disease in this country alone exceed 140 billion dollars a year, and this figure does not include the societal cost of lost productivity — estimated to be 30 billion dollars annually — or the terrible emotional toll that attends the loss of a parent or a spouse.

Great strides have been made in the treatment of heart disease, once it has been detected. In the past ten years, the mortality rate for coronary artery disease, the cause of heart attack, has declined by twenty-two percent. The chance of dying from a heart attack, once a patient has reached the hospital is now less that one in ten.

But in many ways this is a hollow victory. While the death *rate* has dropped, the *incidence* of heart disease continues to increase and the number of people with heart disease continues to grow. It is estimated that in the United States today, 15 million people are afflicted with some form of heart disease.

Medical research continues to advance on many fronts, but as yet the cause of this terrible malady is not known. While we continue to search for clues and pray that prevention will pay off, we have little but early detection to offer the patients who now wait in the ante-room.

CHAPTER 1

NORMAL HEART DEVELOPMENT
AND FUNCTION
What Makes It Tick?

The heart begins its development as a blood vessel which enlarges, twists into an S-shaped loop and partitions itself into four chambers. Within these chambers, four check valves develop to insure that blood flows in only one direction. Each of the four chambers is made of muscle tissue and has the ability to contract, propelling the blood along. By the time an unborn baby is in it's third month of development, the formation of the heart is complete, and it begins to beat.

The heart is essentially a muscular pump, or rather two pumps connected in series, each having a main pumping chamber — the ventricle — and in front of it, a smaller booster pump — the atrium. Blood returning to the heart from the body comes first to the right atrium from which it is pumped through the triscuspid valve, so named for its three leaflets, into the right ventricle. From the right ventricle, blood is pumped through the pulmonary valve into the lungs where it absorbs oxygen and gives off carbon dioxide.

From the lungs this oxygenated blood returns to the left atrium, passing through the mitral valve (named for its resemblance to the pointed bishop's miter hat) and on into the left ventricle which pumps it out through the aortic valve to the body. **(Figure 1)**

With each heartbeat, about half of the blood within the heart, or about four ounces, is pumped forward. This pumping action generates a pressure in the arteries of about 120 mm Hg, the so called systolic blood pressure, or the top number of a blood pressure reading. (The pressure required to raise a column of mercury 120 millimeters) When the heart relaxes between beats, the arterial pressure decreases steadily, while the heart is filling, to a pressure of about 80 mm Hg. This diastolic pressure, the lower number of a blood pressure reading, is the lowest the pressure falls prior to the next heart beat.

FIGURE 1

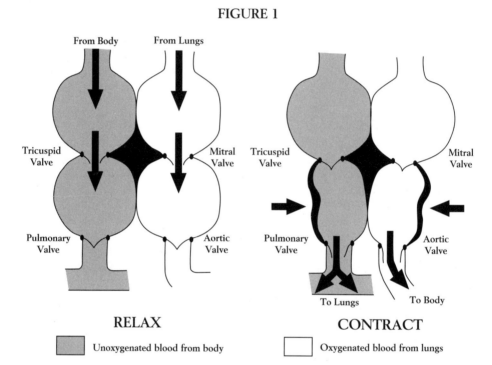

In diastole, the heart relaxes and blood flows into the heart from the body and the lungs. With contraction (systole) tricuspid and mitral valves close to prevent back flow. Pulmonary and aortic valves open to allow blood to leave the heart.

At rest the heart pumps about five quarts of blood a minute, but it can increase its output to nearly forty quarts a minute with extreme exertion such as a trained athlete might experience at the end of a 440-yard dash.

Prior to birth the unborn infant is not breathing, and all of the functions of the lung are supplied by the placenta. Since there is no need for blood to go to the lungs, it is diverted from the right side of the heart to the left side of the heart, bypassing the lungs, through two holes in the septum, or partition, which divide the two sides of the heart. In addition to these two holes, there is a bypass which connects the pulmonary artery with the aorta. Through this connection, any blood which finds its way into the pulmonary artery, passes back into the general circulation without going to the lungs.

Shortly after birth, these two holes and the by-pass close, the short cuts are cut off, and the normal blood flow through the lungs begins. As discussed later, three of the most common forms of congenital heart disease are due to failure of one or more of these short cuts to close.

The normal heart rhythm is maintained by a microscopic natural pacemaker located within the wall of the right atrium. This tiny pacesetter, running on a sort of biologic electricity, spontaneously paces the heart sixty or seventy times a minute. The impulses from this pacemaker are transmitted down through the heart by way of specialized conduction fibers first activating the two atriums and then the two ventricles which contract over and over in response to the stimulation in linked sequence.

Although this natural pacemaker has its own intrinsic rate, it is subject to regulation by outside influences. Stimulation from the vagus nerve can slow the pacing rate, while chemicals such as adrenalin and caffeine can speed it up.

The heart is in the curious position of pumping blood to itself. The blood flow to the heart is supplied by three coronary arteries which originate as branches off the aorta just beyond the heart. These three coronary arteries, in the adult about the size of macaroni, spread down over the surface of the heart muscle, each vessel supplying blood supply and oxygen to about one-third of the heart. This fortunate arrangement limits the amount of heart that can be damaged if one of these vessels becomes occluded. Even so, it is obstruction of these coronary arteries that plagues modern man and accounts for more death and disability than any other disease of any other body part.

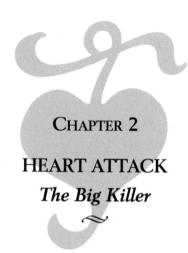

CHAPTER 2

HEART ATTACK
The Big Killer

Heart attacks were first diagnosed in 1912 and since that time have become the largest single killer of Americans. Each year 1.1 million Americans have heart attacks and 30 percent of those die, most within the first few hours.

"Heart attack" is a lay term often used by patients to refer to any type of sudden heart disorder, such as an abnormal heart rhythm or even congestive heart failure. But when doctors use the term, they are referring to damage to the heart caused by blockage of one of the coronary arteries. This heart damage is also known as myocardial infarction or MI.

A heart attack (myocardial infarction) is the end result of a disease of the coronary arteries which results in progressive narrowing or blockage of one or more of the blood vessels that supply blood and oxygen to the heart. The blockage develops slowly over many years, like scale in the cellar pipes, gradually throttling the blood flow. The blockage does not extend the entire length of the affected blood vessel but is limited to a short segment, like a copper pipe crimped with pliers. Beyond the narrowing, the remainder of the blood vessel is usually normal. This segmental nature of coronary disease is the basis for by-pass surgery in which pieces of leg veins are used to "by-pass" the diseased segments. **(Figure 2)**

When the narrowing in the artery reaches a critically small size, blood flow to part of the heart muscle is insufficient and symptoms develop. At first the symptoms — chest pain or pressure or shortness of breath — are present only with exertion such as hurrying or walking uphill or lifting. These exercises cause the heart to need more oxygen or blood supply, but because of the narrowed blood vessel, blood flow cannot be increased to meet the heart's needs and the affected heart muscle, starved for oxygen, aches. With further progression of the narrowing, the blood flow in the diseased vessel is not sufficient, even at rest, and pain can occur with minimal activity.

Heart pain which comes and goes is referred to as angina pectoris [*angina*, pain + *pectoris*, chest], and is a warning sign that one or more of the coronary arteries is partially blocked.

FIGURE 2

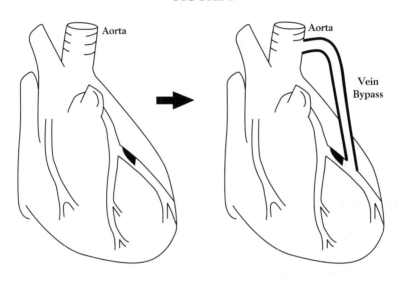

A vein is sewn from the aorta to the coronary artery to "by-pass" the narrowing.

The severity of the symptoms vary from person to person. You would think that a disease that can be fatal would produce severe warning symptoms, like slamming your finger in the car door. But this is not always the case. Some patients do have severe chest pain, but others have shortness of breath, or what they call "pressure" in their chest or a feeling they confuse with "gas" and indigestion. Sometimes the discomfort spreads down one or both arms, into the neck and jaw, or to the back. This variation in symptoms may explain why so many people with coronary artery disease drop dead. Either they do not get a warning, or they do not get the warning they expect.

Thus the danger of coronary artery disease is not related so much to the intensity of the symptoms, but rather what it takes to bring the symptoms on. Chest pain at rest or with minimal activity is a bad sign and usually indicates severe narrowing of at least one coronary artery.

As the narrowing in the coronary artery becomes more severe, the inside of the blood vessel can be reduced to a pinpoint size. The blood flow through this tiny opening becomes so slow that the blood can spontaneously clot, blocking the opening completely and cutting off the blood flow to a part of the heart. If blood flow is not restored promptly, part of the heart dies.

If the heart damage is extensive, there is not enough normal heart muscle left to power the circulation and death comes from heart failure, sometimes during the first few days, but more commonly sometime during the next few months.

The most feared early complication of heart attack is ventricular fibrillation, a fatal rhythm disturbance that can kill in seconds and often occurs early in the course of a heart attack. It is ventricular fibrillation that is the most likely cause of the sudden death, or cardiac arrest, which occurs within the first two hours of the heart attack.

Ventricular fibrillation is an uncontrolled, rapid contraction of the heart. The damaged heart muscle, irritable because of the damage, begins to beat too rapidly for effective pumping, circulation fails, blood pressure falls and death results. Ventricular fibrillation can occur unexpectedly in the early stages of even a "small" heart attack leading to death from a heart attack that by its size would not otherwise be fatal. This is one of the great tragedies of heart attack — that death can, and does occur in patients with hearts "too good to die".

During a heart attack, the greatest danger is within the first two hours. Most of those who are going to die from heart attack do so within the first two hours, usually before arriving at the hospital. For those reaching the hospital, the chance of dying drops to less than ten percent.

> *I can't complain. It's been three months and*
> *I'm already back to playing tennis.*
> Joe — age 87. Heart attack victim.

The treatment of heart attack comes in three stages: emergency care, monitored healing and rehabilitation.

The first order of business is to save the threatened life by stabilizing the heart rhythm, maintaining an adequate blood pressure and doing everything possible to open up the blocked coronary artery that is causing the heart attack.

It is pretty clear now that a heart attack is caused by a blood clot which forms at the site of a partially blocked coronary artery. In the past few years drugs have been developed which can dissolve the blood clot and open up the blocked blood vessel preventing or minimizing heart muscle damage. The earlier that these drugs are given in the course of a heart attack, the more likely they are to dissolve the clot. The sooner the clot is dissolved and the blood flow is restored, the less the heart damage will be.

The beneficial effect of opening the blood vessel falls off rapidly if the drug is given after three to four hours. Therefore it is critical to administer these drugs as early in the course of the heart attack as possible. The longer the blood supply to the heart is cut off, the more heart muscle is damaged. Those providing emergency care to patients with heart attack are driven by this therapeutic approach which can be summarized in one short sentence.

Time is muscle.

These so-called thrombolytic drugs are available in virtually every hospital emergency room in the country. Patients who think they may be having a heart attack should get to the nearest emergency room as soon as possible so that this treatment can begin without delay.

In the second phase of treatment, efforts are centered around monitoring the healing process. Nothing can speed this healing process. It takes time. A broken leg can be put in a cast to rest it while it heals, but the heart can be put at rest only by putting the body at rest. Once, patients were kept in hospital three to six weeks after a heart attack. That much inactivity produced its own problems. Now, heart attack patients are hospitalized five to seven days. By that time, the healing process has gotten a good start and most of the immediate danger period has passed.

During this rest period, when the physician has the patient's undivided attention, is a good time to teach them about heart attack, what they might have done to contribute to it, and what they can do to make sure that it never happens again.

To provide patients recovering from heart attack with the best advice, more information about the condition of their heart is needed. The heart attack from which they have just recovered was caused when one of the three heart blood vessels became blocked and part of the heart supplied by that blood vessel was damaged. The damaged area will heal, like an injury anywhere else in the body. At that point what needs to be done depends on whether or not the two remaining heart blood vessels show any signs of blockage which could lead to further heart damage or leave the patient disabled by angina. (see Chapter 3)

Like an airliner, the body has a lot of built-in redundancy. There are lots of extra parts. There are two eyes, two lungs, two kidneys, and a lot of extra brain. There is also a lot of extra heart muscle, and the arrangement of the coronary blood vessels ordinarily insures that only a third of the heart could be damaged from any one heart attack. Following a heart attack, the damaged part of the heart will heal, and for a middle-aged person that leaves enough normal heart for a normal, active life. The trick is to prevent further damage.

For many years, the prevalent attitude of patients and physicians following a heart attack was one of relief, a feeling that a trying and dangerous episode had passed. But with a better understanding of the treacherous natural history of coronary artery disease, we now know that surviving a heart attack is not only an occasion for relief but also of concern.

A heart attack is not the end but the beginning. A person who has a heart attack has identified himself as someone who has a lethal disease. The heart attack they sustained was the result of occlusion of one of the three coronary arteries. After survival is insured, the main interest shifts to the state of the remaining two coronary arteries. Whether or not the remaining vessels are diseased (and, if so, how much) will determine what the rest of the person's life will be like and to some extent how long it might be.

Evaluation of the patient after a heart attack should proceed with the same devotion as would be directed to a patient who coughs up blood. The proper response is not only, "Well, I'm sure glad it stopped," but also, "Where did THAT come from?"

Physicians learned the hard way that the standard electrocardiogram (EKG) is not a very good predictor of future heart attack. Unfortunately, some of those stories about patients dropping dead after having a normal EKG are true. In an effort to improve the predictive accuracy of the EKG, the stress test was developed. It is based on the assumption that stressing the heart might show trouble that was not apparent at rest, much like taking your car out on the interstate. Therefore before sending a heart attack patient home from the hospital, it is customary to perform a stress test in an effort to detect any trouble with the remaining arteries.

The standard treadmill exercise test proved to be much better at detecting coronary artery disease than the resting EKG. Patients are exercised on a treadmill and the EKG is examined for characteristic changes, not present at rest, that might indicate the presence of coronary artery disease.

However it soon became apparent that the treadmill exercise test had its own limitations. Since the test depends on a change from a normal to an abnormal EKG with exercise, the test is of little value if the EKG at rest is abnormal. In addition some patients, particularly women for some reason, have abnormal stress tests when no coronary artery disease is present. Also some stress tests are negative in patients who have coronary artery disease.

In the 1980s, the thallium scan, or myocardial perfusion scan, was developed in an attempt to improve on the predictive accuracy of the treadmill stress test. Thallium, a radioactive isotope with a very short half-life, is absorbed by the heart muscle in proportion to the amount of blood flow it receives. Since thallium is radioactive, it can be detected by a special x-ray camera.

For this test patients are exercised on a treadmill to increase the heart blood flow as much as possible. At peak exercise thallium, or a similar isotope such as technetium, is injected into an arm vein and pictures of the heart are made immediately after exercise and again three hours later. By comparing these two sets of pictures, it is possible to tell if the heart circulation is normal, if the heart has been damaged, or if parts of the heart are in jeopardy.

In the normal heart all the coronary arteries are open and blood flow and isotope uptake by the heart are uniform. The resulting heart images appear as a homogeneous white ball. If there is blockage in one of the heart arteries, the blood flow to the part of the heart supplied by that diseased vessel is reduced, the amount of isotope that is taken up by that part of the heart is reduced, and this defect appears as a black, PAC-MAN-like bite out of the ordinarily round, white heart image.

If that part of the heart is permanently damaged from a completely blocked coronary artery that has caused a heart attack, the defect present immediately after exercise will persist even at the time of the second set of pictures three hours later.

However if the defect detected immediately after exercise is produced by partial blockage of a blood vessel, the defect will be filled in on the later pictures by thallium which has gradually seeped by the narrowing into the heart muscle. In this way isotope scanning can distinguish between heart muscle that has been damaged by a completely occluded, or blocked, blood vessel and heart muscle that is threatened by a partially occluded one.

The isotope scan greatly improved a physician's ability to detect coronary artery disease, and tens of thousands of these exams are performed each year. It is considerably more accurate than the standard treadmill, but is considerably more trouble and more expensive. Sometimes a treadmill test is all that is required, and if it provides the information needed there is no reason to proceed to a isotope scan. However in many cases the increased accuracy is required and is worth the extra trouble and expense. Since the treadmill test is designed to detect changes from a normal resting EKG to an abnormal EKG with exercise, the isotope scan is most helpful when the resting EKG is abnormal or when the results of the treadmill test are equivocal.

If partially blocked blood vessels are detected, further treatment may be required to prevent those vessels from blocking completely and causing further damage. If no additional risk from partially blocked blood vessels is detected, the patient's future will be determined by how much heart muscle was damaged by the heart attack. If the damage was minimal — from blockage of one of the smaller heart blood vessels — the patient can look forward to a normal life style. If the damage was extensive, as would result from blockage of one of the major heart blood vessels or from the cumulative result of several heart attacks, the heart muscle may be weakened to the point that it can no longer support the body's needs for blood flow and the syndrome of congestive heart failure develops. This is discussed further in Chapter 8 .

Strictly speaking there is no such thing as a "small" heart attack. It is true that the less heart damage the better, but use of the word "small" implies a false sense of security that, unfortunately, patients and their families tend to fix on. Even a "small" heart attack can be fatal if it causes a lethal heart rhythm disturbance like ventricular fibrillation.

The amount of heart damaged by a heart attack depends on two factors — the size of the blocked blood vessel and the length of time the blockage persists. If the blockage persists and the blocked blood vessel is small, the amount of damage will be small. However, a "small" amount of damage can also result if a major blood vessel is blocked transiently. This can occur if the blood clot blocking the vessel dissolves, allowing blood flow to be restored before much damage has had time to occur. If this happens — transient blockage in a large blood vessel — the amount of heart damage may be limited, but this is little cause for comfort. Unless something is done to relieve — or by-pass — the original severe narrowing, an obstructing blood clot may form again; and, if persistent, the amount of future heart damage could be extensive

Therefore, the concept of "small" heart attack can be misleading. Rather than serving as a source of relief, a "small" heart attack should direct attention to the cause and efforts to prevent a potentially disastrous recurrence.

Following a heart attack, patients who have normal stress tests are advised to have periodic stress tests to monitor the condition of their coronary arteries to detect trouble as soon as possible before any further heart damage occurs.

If a normal stress test becomes abnormal, there are two possible courses of action. If the goal is to control symptoms, treatment with medicine can be used. Medical treatment often controls the symptoms of chest pain and shortness of breath, but as far as we know it does nothing to relieve the blood vessel blockage which usually progresses. If the goal is to try to prolong life, more information is needed.

Whether coronary artery disease is dangerous or disabling depends on exactly which blood vessel or vessels are affected, how many are affected, and to what extent they are affected. If a small blood vessel is partially blocked, not much heart muscle would be damaged if it became occluded, and the risk, therefore, would be relatively small. If, however, the partial blockage involves a large blood vessel, the risk is considerably higher since complete blockage of a large coronary artery could cause more extensive heart damage. The risk is further increased if several coronary arteries are affected.

It is very difficult to tell from the exercise test alone whether or not the coronary disease is dangerous and further study is required to clarify the diagnosis, determine the risk, and plan the best management to minimize it.

The isotope scan does not show the actual blood vessels themselves. It shows only whether or not there is equal blood flow to all parts of the heart. A reduced blood flow to one part of the heart implies that there is a narrowing in the vessel supplying that area, but to know exactly which blood vessels and how many, the vessels need to be visualized directly.

The coronary arteries that we need to see do not show up on ordinary x-ray and a coronary angiogram [*angio*, blood vessel + *gram*, a record] is required. In this technique, an x-ray dye is injected directly into the coronary arteries and as the dye passes down the artery it outlines the blood vessel, and the blockages can be clearly identified, much as a stomach ulcer can be outlined by the dye swallowed during a stomach x-ray.

The difficulty with a coronary angiogram is getting the dye to the coronary arteries. We don't need to see all the blood vessels in the body, only the coronary arteries. To get the dye to the coronaries it must enter the arterial circulation. The usual route is by way of the large blood vessel in the groin (femoral artery). This blood vessel is about the size of an index finger and is about a quarter of an inch under the skin.

At the time of a coronary angiogram, the skin of the groin is anesthetized and a needle is introduced through the skin into the artery. Next a small, flexible guide wire is introduced through the needle, and then a small catheter, about the size of a ballpoint pen refill and about three feet long, is advanced over the guide wire into the artery. The guide wire is then removed leaving the catheter tip inside the artery.

The femoral arteries from each leg join together to form the aorta which is about the size of a broomstick and this vessel, in turn, connects to the heart. The small soft flexible catheter can be advanced back up through this large aorta to the heart under fluoroscopic guidance. When the tip of the catheter is in the right position, a small amount of dye can be injected directly into the coronary artery and motion picture photographs can be made.

The angiogram is usually completed within fifteen to twenty minutes, discomfort is minimal, and general anesthesia is not required. Ordinarily only a mild tranquilizer is used to allay some of the anxiety.

Eight or ten sets of movie pictures are made, the catheter is removed, and pressure is held on the puncture site in the groin till the vessel naturally seals off. There is no incision, and there are no stitches. After the puncture wound has sealed off, the patients are kept in bed for several hours to avoid activity which might break the seal in the artery and allow bleeding under the skin. If this occurs it is not serious, but it can produce a painful bruise in the groin, and a few hours of bedrest is all that is required to prevent this.

This rest period allows the cardiologist who performed the angiogram to develop the films and review them carefully. Prior to discharge, the cardiologist meets with the patient to explain what was found, what it means, and what the choices are.

If the angiogram shows that there is minimal coronary disease with a low risk, medicine is usually the best treatment. However if several arteries are involved and the risk of heart attack is high, sometimes coronary artery by-pass surgery is the only treatment which will be effective. Occasionally the disease process is so extensive that the risk of surgery is prohibitive. If only one or two vessels are involved, the obstructions can sometimes be removed with angioplasty and surgery can be avoided.

A few years ago there were few treatment options for patients with coronary artery disease. Now there are too many choices. The problem we have now is not so much trying to decide who needs treatment, but trying to match up the patient's condition with the best possible treatment option.

The risk of complications during a coronary angiogram is nearly zero, but it is not zero, and there is a long list of terrible things that can happen during an angiogram such as heart attack, stroke, heart rhythm disturbances, blood clots, hemorrhage and even death. But the chance of one of these things happening to the average person is exceedingly low. If, in the physician's judgement, the information is needed to best plan a patient's treatment, the small risk of an angiogram is more than offset by the potential benefits.

Coronary angiography is not a new test. It has been performed since the 1960s. Once performed only at large medical centers, coronary angiography is now done in over 1600 hospitals throughout the country. During the past thirty-five years, great effort has been directed toward anticipating and preventing complications. Catheterization laboratories, equipped like intensive care units, are prepared to deal with complications if they should arise.

Most of the complications of angiography occur in the people you might expect, the elderly and those with far-advanced heart disease. Taking all comers, the risk of dying during coronary angiography is about 1 in 100,000. But the risks of angiography must be balanced against not doing the catheterization and trying to manage a patient with a deadly disease on the basis of inadequate information. It's not that one way is safe and the other dangerous. There is a risk either way. What physicians are looking for is the safest way out of a bad situation. The risk of doing coronary angiography must be balanced against the risk of not doing it. If the risk cannot be justified then the angiography should not be done.

Patients should not have a coronary angiogram just because the doctor says so. It is the doctor's job to make sure that the patient understands the risks and benefits of either course of action. The patient must make the decision to have the angiogram, not because the doctor says so, but because the patient is convinced that it is the right thing to do.

For some patients, especially those with severely diseased coronary arteries, by-pass surgery is the best treatment we have to offer. The risk of dying during coronary artery by-pass surgery in most centers is less that two percent and most of this risk is accounted for by patients who are older, who have associated lung and kidney trouble. Otherwise healthy, young patients have an extremely low risk. Ordinarily following surgery, patients are up in the hall on the third day, go home on the fifth day, and depending on their job, can return to work and a normal life within a few weeks. This contrasts sharply with the early days of by-pass surgery when patients were kept in the hospital after surgery for several weeks.

Balloon angioplasty [*angio*, vessel + *plasty*, to mold] is often the best treatment for severe narrowing of one coronary artery, particularly if the artery is a large one and the heart attack caused by its occlusion would be extensive.

During angioplasty, which is also performed in the catheterization laboratory, a long catheter with a small balloon on the tip is threaded up the arteries from the leg into the diseased coronary artery. When the balloon is in the correct position at the site of the partial blockage, it is inflated and flattens the obstructing material against the wall of the vessel. **(Figure 3)**

The risk of angioplasty is much less than that for by-pass surgery. The main risk at the time of angioplasty is that during the attempt to dilate the narrowed blood vessel it can be ruptured. If this occurs, emergency by-pass surgery is required. To deal with this possibility, cardiac surgeons are on stand-by for every angioplasty procedure so that surgery can be performed immediately if needed. The chance of rupturing a blood vessel during angioplasty is about two percent in most centers and the expected mortality of emergency by-pass surgery is about two percent, so the risk of dying as the result of angioplasty is roughly two percent of two percent, or about 4 in 10,000. This very low risk is one of the attractive features of angioplasty and it is often the preferred approach when the coronary artery anatomy is suitable.

FIGURE 3

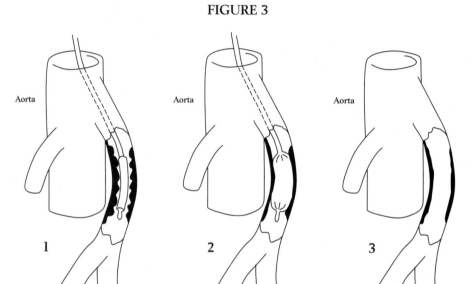

Balloon tip of angioplasty catheter is inflated in the coronary artery compressing the plaque and opening the vessel.

The biggest drawback, by far, to angioplasty is that it sometimes has to be repeated. After being successfully dilated the blood vessel can again become occluded. If this happens, it is usually within the first two or three months and repeat angioplasty is required. The rationale for repeating the procedure is based on the disease process.

The original plaque which occluded the vessel required several years to develop and is composed of crusty and sometimes calcified material. On the other hand, the plaque which forms in the first few months after angioplasty is composed of a soft, soapy material, very easy to dilate, and the second dilatation is almost always successful. Redilatation is required in as many as twenty-five percent of patients undergoing angioplasty; but as undesirable as this is, it is still successful in a majority of patients and relieves them of the symptoms and danger of coronary artery disease that would otherwise require by-pass surgery which has a much higher risk.

Recently, in an effort to reduce the number of angioplasties that have to be re-done, the technique has been altered. After the vessel is dilated, a small stent, or mesh tube, is placed in the vessel using the same catheter used to perform the angioplasty. This stent acts like a tiny culvert to support the sides of the vessel and prevent blockage from developing. In some patients, the obstructing material can be scraped away using a small blade attached to the catheter. This procedure is called atherectomy [*atheroma*, the obstructing plaque + *ectomy*, to remove]. Both stents and atherectomy have improved the results of angioplasty.

A heart attack is a very stressful illness psychologically. In the wake of a heart attack, patients pass through several stages of adjustment. Typically the initial reaction to a heart attack is denial. "This can't be happening to me!" Following this denial phase, there is a period of anger and hostility. Patients feel that somehow they have been singled out. Once the anger has subsided there is often a period of depression as the impact sinks in, and the patient realizes that the illness which they have just sustained might have very well killed them. This feeling of vulnerability is new to many and often very unsettling.

Ordinarily each of these phases last only a few days, but some patients never get beyond the denial, or the hostility, or the depression and this failure to adjust can interfere significantly with their rehabilitation and the resumption of a normal life.

Psychological counseling, in addition to that provided by the patient's physician, is sometimes required; but often the best reassurance is a thorough, systematic evaluation which can reassure the patient that either the coronary arteries are normal and there is little likelihood of further trouble or that further trouble has been detected and is being dealt with.

CHAPTER 3

ANGINA

What Is It and Why is My Doctor So Concerned?

A ngina is a confusing term. Taken from the Latin *angina pectoris* meaning pain in the chest, it has been used to refer both to the pain caused by coronary artery disease and to the condition itself. Angina is caused by a narrowing of one or more of the coronary arteries. This process, which takes years to develop, gradually narrows a segment of one or more coronary arteries limiting the blood flow to a part of the heart. In the beginning the flow limitation is not significant, and no symptoms are present, but with time the narrowing becomes more severe, blood flow is limited and symptoms develop.

Symptoms usually occur first during exercise. If the narrowing is not severe, the heart has adequate blood flow and oxygen at rest. With exertion the heart needs more blood supply, but because of the narrowing which acts as a throttle, part of the heart can't get adequate oxygen and it aches. With rest the demand for oxygen decreases and the pain subsides. This exertional chest pain is characteristic of coronary artery disease. In time, the narrowing can become so severe and the blood flow to the heart so limited that pain occurs with excitement or emotional stress or even during sleep. Therefore it is not the severity of the pain that is an indicator of the danger, but what it takes to bring it on.

Pain at rest or with minimal exertion usually indicates severe narrowing of one or more of the coronary arteries. At this stage, the blood flow through the pin-point opening is very sluggish and even a tiny blood clot can block off the vessel completely causing a heart attack.

Thus the same process that causes angina can eventually cause a heart attack, and this is why doctors are so concerned when patients develop angina. Angina is not only discomfort, interfering with activities, but it is also a warning sign that there is heart blood vessel trouble and that a heart attack may be imminent. Angina can be disabling, but it can also kill. However, it is not the severity of the pain that is an accurate indicator of the the danger, but what it takes to bring it on.

Angina is a treacherous disease. You would expect that the symptoms caused by a disease that could kill you would be real attention-getters, but often this is not the case. The pain itself may not be that severe, and this sometimes leads patients to be too tolerant. The key is that, at least in the beginning, the discomfort is almost always related to exertion — brought on by effort and relieved by rest.

In the past there was not much to do for angina except restrict the patient's activities to avoid the pain. They simply sat and waited to die. Now there are too many choices. The trick is to match up the trouble with the proper treatment. What treatment is required depends on the nature and extent of the coronary artery disease. Some patients need medicine. Some need by-pass surgery. Some need balloon angioplasty. Patients who can be treated with medicine do not need surgery and vice versa.

But there is hope here. Angina is not necessarily a death sentence. Nowadays, if we can get at it early enough, coronary artery disease can almost always be fixed — one way or another — and patients can look forward to getting back to doing pretty much what they please. The important thing is to get at it early before blockage of one of the heart arteries has damaged the heart beyond repair. Until there is an effective prevention, early detection is the key.

If the pain from angina is due to partial blockage in a small blood vessel, the risk may be relatively low. In this case, if the partial blockage progresses to complete blockage the amount of heart damaged by this heart attack would be relatively small.

However, if the pain is due to partial blockage in a major blood vessel, the risk is high since occlusion of this major vessel would damage so much of the heart that survival is unlikely.

It is very difficult to tell from looking at the outside of someone whether the angina which they are experiencing is dangerous or merely painful. Stress testing can confirm the presence of coronary artery disease but it is limited in its ability to clarify the extent of the disease or accurately predict the risk. For this, a coronary angiogram [*angio*, blood vessel + *gram*, a record] is required.

During this procedure, usually performed on an outpatient basis, a small catheter is introduced into a blood vessel in the groin through the skin which has been anesthetized. The catheter is advanced to the heart where x-ray dye is injected into the coronary arteries and photographs of the arteries can be made. Any areas of blockage can be demonstrated.

The main value of a coronary angiogram is that the anatomy of the coronary arteries can be visualized directly. It is possible to see which arteries and how many are involved and how extensive the process is. After this — and only after this — can a patient's risk be defined and the treatment intelligently planned. If you had one thing which would determine pretty much what the rest of your life would be like and how long it might be, it would be a coronary angiogram.

If the risk of heart attack is low and relief of pain is the goal of treatment, many good drugs are available. If the coronary anatomy is threatening, angioplasty [*angio*, blood vessel + *plasty*, to mold] to open the vessel or open heart surgery to by-pass it may be required.

Medical treatment, angioplasty and by-pass surgery are not necessarily alternatives or options for every patient, and it is difficult to compare overall results. Each is a treatment of a different condition. Some patients have conditions that are best treated with medicine, others with angioplasty and others have conditions best treated with by-pass surgery. Patients who need angioplasty and patients who need by-pass surgery are different patients, with different problems.

For example, appendectomy and cholecystectomy are both valuable, time-proven procedures. If you have appendicitis you need an appendectomy. If you have gallbladder disease you need a cholecystectomy. You would not recommend an appendectomy for someone with gall bladder disease. You would not recommend medicine or angioplasty if by-pass surgery is what was needed.

Angioplasty is most commonly performed on patients with disease involving one or two of the coronary arteries. Nearly 500,000 of these procedures were performed last year. In this procedure a small catheter with a deflated balloon attached to the tip is threaded up through the leg blood vessel and down the partially-blocked coronary artery. No surgery or general anesthesia is required. When the deflated balloon is astride the area of blockage, the balloon is inflated stretching the narrowing, opening up the artery and restoring normal blood flow. (Figure 3, see page 14) Symptoms are relieved immediately and patients go home and back to work the following day.

Atherectomy [*atheroma*, the obstructing plaque + *ectomy*, to remove] is similar to angioplasty except rather than dilating the narrowing with a balloon, a small cutting device is used to pare away and remove the obstructing material. In some patients, tiny mesh tubes called stents are placed in the vessel to support the walls after angioplasty or atherectomy.

Much has been written in the popular press about the shortcomings of both angioplasty, atherectomy and stent placement. There are the same cries of uselessness and abuse that were leveled — for a while — at coronary by-pass surgery. But no one any longer seriously doubts the value and efficacy of by-pass surgery as a procedure. It would be immoral now to deny bypass surgery to patients who might benefit solely for the purpose of studying comparative results. Those studies were done and will not be repeated. Is by-pass a perfect operation? No. It is always successful? No. Does everyone with coronary disease need it? No. Is it helpful for those who need it? No question.

The same is true for angioplasty and atherectomy. In twenty percent of cases, the procedure has to be redone, usually within the first three months.. Reocclusion, if it is going to happen usually does so within that time. If reocclusion does occur after angioplasty, the treatment is repeated, and this second dilitation is almost always successful. The reason for this is as follows.

At the time of the first angioplasty, the obstructing plaque is often hard, calcified material which has been building up in the artery for twenty to thirty years. However, when the vessel becomes blocked after angioplasty the obstructing material, which develops much more quickly, is usually a soft, soapy cheesy material, more like wax than chalk and dilitation or removal of this material is usually much easier. Hence the rationale for the repeat procedure. Otherwise you might be inclined to say if it didn't work the first time, why do it again? The fact is that it did work the first time. The reocclusion just requires re-treatment and experience has born out the wisdom of this approach.

Also keep in mind that reocclusion only develops in about twenty percent of cases. This means that eighty percent of the time, the procedure is successful the first time and that no further treatment is required. That the critics in the press focus on the reocclusion only manifests their preoccupation with a man-bites dog story.

> *If I hadn't had the treatment, I wouldn't be here*
> *today. I do everything I want to do. And my wife*
> *doesn't follow me around any more.*
> Jake — age 75. Angioplasty patient

Coronary artery by-pass surgery was developed in the 1960s nearly simultaneously at medical centers in Houston and Cleveland based largely on the success of this type of surgery for treatment of blockage of larger blood vessels in the leg. Each year in the United States alone, some 600,000 coronary artery by-pass operations are performed. The rationale for this operation is based on the fact that the blockage in the coronary arteries is not throughout the length of it, but rather confined to a short segment, like a copper tube crimped with pliers.

During the by-pass operation, the chest cavity is opened and the heart is exposed. A short section of vein — usually from the leg — is removed and one end is attached to the aorta above the heart. The other end of the vein is draped down over the heart and attached to the coronary artery beyond the blockage, bypassing it and restoring normal blood flow to that part of the heart that was "fuel starved". (Figure 2, see page 5) The obstructing material is not removed, but left in place. Early attempts to surgically remove the plaque blocking the artery proved unsuccessful.

Removing the vein from the leg is of little consequence. There is a dual set of veins in the leg, and if one is removed, the other enlarges and takes over the function of both.

Time has proven the value of the by-pass operation in the treatment of coronary artery disease — for those who need it. It is not a perfect operation. There are very definite risks involved and these risks must be weighed against the possible benefits in each patient, a judgment a physician must make with almost any type of treatment. Coronary artery by-pass is not a magic cure-all for coronary artery disease, but it is effective. It can relieve anginal pain, and it is one of the few procedures at our disposal that can prolong life. Perhaps soon something better will come along. Perhaps soon an effective method of preventing coronary disease will be discovered. In the mean time, coronary disease is a crippler and a killer and something must be done for the patients who now wait in the ante room.

Sometimes angina recurs in patients who have had coronary artery by-pass operations. Sometimes this is because, for some reason, the initial operation was technically inadequate. With current surgical skills so excellent and so widespread, technical failure is not common.

Sometimes recurrence of angina is due to closure of one of the venous by-pass grafts. In many cases this occurs because one of the vessels being by-passed, though needing by-pass, was not ideal for by-passing. In these cases, at the time of the operation, the surgeon grafts this "marginal" vessel in addition to the other more suitable ones in the hope that, even though not ideal, the graft will be helpful. When such grafts later fail there is little lost since without the attempt, the diseased vessel would continue to cause trouble. That one of several grafts fails is not an indictment of the operation or the need for it. It is merely the reflection of the infallibility of the surgeon's judgment made under difficult circumstances. And if one of several grafts fails, the patient is usually still better off than without surgery since grafting of the other diseased vessels is effective. The patient with multi-vessel disease has been converted to a patient with single vessel disease, a condition with much less risk and one which is much easier to treat medically.

In other patients, angina which recurs after by-pass surgery is not due to a "failure" of the operation at all but to the subsequent development of obstruction in a vessel which was not diseased at the time of the operation. Which of these several possibilities is the cause of recurrent angina following by-pass can only be determined by coronary angiography.

When possible, rather that using leg veins for the by-pass grafts, the surgeon can use one, or occasionally both, of the internal mammary arteries. These blood vessels — fortunately just the right size and length for grafting — run down along the underside of the rib cage near the breast bone, conveniently near the heart. When used for by-pass grafts the end of the vessel is freed up and plugged into the diseased coronary artery beyond the blockage. The other end of the internal mammary artery remains attached to the aorta at it's original position. These internal mammary artery grafts are particularly successful — perhaps because the artery-to-artery graft is more natural — and most surgeons prefer to use them whenever possible.

CHAPTER 4

HEART RHYTHM DISTURBANCES

Doctor, What Does It Mean When My Heart Skips and Races?

Sometimes the heart rhythm is disturbed as a result of a serious underlying heart condition. Sometimes heart rhythm disturbances develop in hearts that are otherwise perfectly normal. The issue, for the doctor and the patient, is to avoid confusing these two situations.

In many patients with heart rhythm disturbances, no abnormality of the heart can be detected, even after a thorough evaluation. Obviously, something is wrong, usually within the heart's tiny pacemaker, but it is so insignificant that often it can not be detected even on examination of the heart at autopsy, and it is perfectly compatible with a long and active life.

In the heart, as in other parts of the body, it is possible to have a functional disorder without there being a serious structural disorder as the cause of it. For example, every patient with a headache does not have a brain tumor. Every patient with a stomach ache does not have an ulcer. Some conditions like migraine headache and the flu can certainly cause troublesome symptoms; and while they can ruin your day, they are not likely to do you in. It is important, however, to investigate all of these complaints thoroughly to distinguish between the two, so that those with serious conditions can be diagnosed and dealt with and those without them can be reassured.

Heart rhythm disturbances are of two general types and have been classified as atrial or ventricular, based on the site of origin of the rhythm disturbance.

As a rule, atrial arrhythmias are of little serious consequence. On the other hand, ventricular arrhythmias can be more serious and are sometimes life threatening. Atrial and ventricular rhythm disturbances are easily distinguished based on their characteristic changes on the electrocardiogram. However, rhythm disturbances of either type are often transient and between episodes the electrocardiogram, like the EEG (electroencephalogram or brain wave test) between epileptic seizures, may be completely normal. It is important, therefore, for proper identification, to "catch them at it" and record an electrocardiogram during a typical episode. A number of techniques are available to assist in this.

Supraventricular arrhythmias (SVAs), or atrial arrhythmias, originate in or near the pacemaker in the right atrium, the upper chamber of the heart. There are several theories of the origin of SVA but it is simplest — if not most accurate — to think of SVA as originating in an irritable focus in the atrium, much as epileptic seizures originate in an irritable focus in the brain.

The heart, like the brain, runs on a sort of biological electricity. Sometimes stray currents or shorts can occur, causing an extra heart beat. These extra beats are often not felt, but result in a pause, or a resetting of the pacemaker. After the pause, during which the heart is distended with blood, the next beat is more forceful, and it is this forceful beat which is perceived by the patient. Palpitation is a term sometimes used to describe the sensation of skipped or irregular heart beats. Since each heartbeat generates a pulse — which can be felt most easily in the arteries in the neck or at the wrist — these extra beats also cause an irregular pulse. The extra beats and the irregular pulse are not separate disorders but different manifestations of the same disorder.

Occasionally these extra beats can set off a chain reaction, much as a mouse trap tossed into a room full of cocked mouse traps. This chain reaction can cause a sustained rapid heart beat, or tachycardia, which can cause a sensation of the heart racing. Most often, in otherwise normal hearts, this is merely an unpleasant sensation, but can sometimes, if sustained, be associated with a feeling of faintness or weakness or shortness of breath.

It is important to emphasize that this rapid heart action does not damage the heart in any way. The heart loves to go fast. You can not pick up a health magazine these days without reading how important it is to go out and exercise to make the heart go fast. On the other hand, high pressure will ruin the heart. The heart hates high pressure, but it loves to go fast.

For reasons which we do not understand, some individuals are prone to heart rhythm disturbances. The natural history of supraventricular tachycardias can be extremely variable. Sometimes the episodes of tachycardia begin in childhood and continue throughout life. Sometimes the episodes do not begin until adult life and may last a short time or may wax and wane for years. Some patients have only an occasional episode, and others are troubled daily. Still others have frequent episodes of tachycardia for days only to have them to stop completely forever or recur at unpredictable intervals.

Supraventricular arrhythmias can, in sensitive individuals, be set off by extraneous things such as too much alcohol (I have a colleague who can get tachycardia after one drink), coffee, tea, fear, anxiety or fatigue. Different patients have noticed different inciting events and have learned to steer clear of them. In some patients, the tachycardia can be due to a previously unsuspected overactive thyroid — President Bush had this problem — and this should always be investigated in patients presenting with tachycardias.

Usually the episodes of tachycardia are of little consequence, especially in those without underlying heart disease, unless overreacted to emotionally by physicians or patients. Patients — children and adults alike — who have symptomatic arrythmias should be encouraged to lead as normal a life as possible, avoiding only those things which experience has taught them might precipitate the tachycardia.

If symptoms are recurrent and troublesome, medicine may be required to control the tachycardia. Modern physicians don't like to limit patients unnecessarily. We don't like to say, "You have to learn to live with it." If the tachycardia is interfering with a normal life style, it's our job to adjust the medicine so that patients can live a normal life and with the drugs we have today, this is almost always possible.

For those with symptoms which cannot be controlled by medication, a procedure known as ablation is available and may soon be the treatment of choice for supraventricular arrhythmias. In this procedure, a small catheter is threaded up a vein into the heart where, by analyzing recordings made from the catheter tip, the irritable focus can be identified. Once located, this microscopic focus can be destroyed using radiofrequency energy, and the tachycardia can be cured. This painless procedure is performed in the catheterization laboratory in a few minutes and no anaesthesia is required.

The symptoms of supraventricular tachycardia include an awareness of rapid heart beat, usually described as a pounding or fluttering in the chest, and sometimes, if the tachycardia is prolonged, weakness, sweating or faintness. For some patients, these symptoms of supraventricular tachycardia can be alarming, especially when the attacks first begin, and it is sometimes difficult to reassure them that these symptoms which are so frightening are not a sign of some heart disease that will disable them or shorten their lives. Even after a thorough evaluation has excluded any serious problems, reassurance is required. "I wish you didn't have this," I tell them, "and I don't mind you being mad about it, but I don't want you to be afraid."

Atrial fibrillation is one form of supraventricular tachycardia that does pose a special risk. In this condition, the atrium is not contracting but is merely quivering. Since it is not contracting, the atrium does not empty properly, and the blood flow within the atrium can become"stagnant." Blood is a little like Jello, and when the flow slows, it can congeal. In the fibrillating atrium, when the blood flow is abnormal, small blood clots can form and later be released and go to the brain — causing a stroke — or damage one of the other vital organs. To prevent this, blood thinners are recommended, most commonly Coumadin, but in some cases aspirin seems to be adequate. Thus the danger in atrial fibrillation is that it may go untreated. With proper anticoagulation, the danger of stroke is virtually eliminated.

Atrial fibrillation can sometimes be converted back to a regular rhythm using electrical cardioversion. For this procedure, the patient is given an intravenous anesthetic, such as pentothal, and while asleep, an electric current is passed throughout the chest. The current stops the fibrillation, allowing the normal pacing sequence to resume. Since the patients are asleep, no discomfort is involved and once fully awake (usually within a few minutes) the patients can return home. For patients who cannot be successfully treated with medicine, cardioversion is sometimes recommended. This is particularly useful in patients with underlying heart disease who depend on the extra boost which atrial contraction provides to the weakened heart.

Arrhythmias can also originate in the ventricles of the heart. The most common ventricular arrhythmia is the premature ventricular contraction, or PVC. These extra beats can, and often do, occur in perfectly normal people and in these cases are harmless. After a thorough evaluation to exclude underlying heart disease, only reassurance is required. Sometimes, however, PVCs can be an indication of a serious heart condition, usually coronary artery disease.

A more serious ventricular arrhythmia, ventricular tachycardia, occurs when an abnormal "pacemaker" in the ventricle drives the heart at rates which may exceed 250 beats per minute. Since these beats originate in the ventricle rather than the atrium, the usual contraction sequence is not present and the efficient pumping action of the heart is compromised — especially if there is associated disease of the heart valves or the coronary arteries. In this case, the blood pressure can fall to a dangerously low level and the patient may lose consciousness. Ventricular tachycardia, in all cases, is a serious rhythm disturbance and demands immediate investigation.

Ventricular tachycardia can deteriorate to the most feared of all heart rhythm disturbances — ventricular fibrillation. This is to be distinguished from *atrial* fibrillation which is usually of little consequence. With ventricular fibrillation, the ventricle, the main pumping chamber of the heart, does not contract, but merely quivers, and the circulation stops.

If not interrupted, usually by electrical defibrillation (the "paddles" seen on television shows), ventricular fibrillation is always fatal. At times ventricular fibrillation can occur spontaneously, without preceding ventricular tachycardia. This is the fatal rhythm that develops in the early stages of a heart attack and is responsible for most cases of sudden death. Cardiopulmonary resuscitation can sustain a person with ventricular fibrillation for a short time, especially if applied promptly, but for survival, defibrillation is required.

Especially in patients with ventricular arrhythmias, it is an important issue to identify and treat the underlying heart condition. Most often this is coronary artery disease. Lack of proper blood supply makes the ventricle particularly irritable and susceptible to arrhythmias. Often treating the coronary artery disease will prevent further trouble from ventricular rhythm disturbances.

For those in whom it is not possible to treat the underlying heart condition, a number of effective drugs are available for the treatment of the rhythm disturbance itself. As with supraventricular arrhythmias, diligence is required to find the right drugs or dosage which is effective. To assist in this process of drug selection electrophysiologic studies are sometimes required.

Electrophysiologic studies, or EPS, are done in the catheterization laboratory. Using special catheters threaded into the ventricular chamber, the heart is stimulated electrically in an attempt to induce the arrhythmia. The patients are sedated, and electrical defibrillators are immediately available to terminate the ventricular arrhythmia when it is produced. After inducing the arrhythmia, a series of drugs is given, one after another and the procedure is repeated until a drug is found which can prevent the arrhythmia. In this way an effective treatment can be found quickly rather than through a long series of drug trials as an outpatient, during which time the patient is unprotected if the agent being tried is not effective.

For patients for whom no effective drug can be found, or for patients who have troublesome drug side effects, implantable automatic defibrillators are available. These instruments, placed under the skin, can detect a ventricular arrhythmia if it occurs, and terminate it with a pre-programed electric shock.

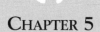

CHAPTER 5

HEART VALVE DISEASE

Did Anyone Ever Tell You That You Had A Heart Murmur?

A heart murmur is just a noise and having a heart murmur does not necessarily mean that you have heart trouble.

The heart is a pump with four one-way valves. The intake valves (mitral on the left and tricuspid on the right) open to allow the heart to fill. They close when the heart contracts to prevent the blood from going backward. The outlet valves (the pulmonic on the right and the aortic on the left) open when the heart contracts to allow the blood to flow out to the lungs and the body and close when the heart relaxes to fill so the blood will not flow back into the heart. (Figure 1, see page 2)

When the heart contracts and pumps blood the "LUB-DUP" sound that the heart makes is caused by the closing of the heart valves. The "LUB" is produced by the closing of the intake valves and the "DUP" produced by the closing of the outlet valves. The valves make no noise when they open.

Ordinarily it is not possible to hear the movement of the blood, but in some young, healthy individuals, the circulation is so brisk that turbulence is created as the blood flows through perfectly normal valves. This turbulence creates a liquid, pulsing "swish" sound which can be heard with a stethoscope and this noise is called a murmur.

In these patients, usually children, there is no evidence of valve abnormality and these murmurs are called, for want of a better name, "innocent" heart murmurs. These murmurs almost always disappear in adult life and are of no consequence except for the anxiety they cause among concerned parents.

Heart murmurs can also be caused by abnormalities of the heart valves, or by congenital heart defects, as discussed in Chapter 10. A thorough investigation can determine the origin of the murmur and whether or not it is "innocent" or due to a structural abnormality.

An abnormal heart valve can cause a murmur in one of two ways. A valve which does not close properly can leak and the leakage can cause a murmur. A valve which is partially blocked (or stenotic) can cause a murmur by partially obstructing the normal blood flow. If the murmur occurs when the heart contracts, it is referred to as a systolic murmur. If the murmur occurs when the heart is filling, it is called a diastolic murmur.

A narrowing in the aortic or the pulmonic valve (outlet valves) can cause a systolic heart murmur by creating turbulence as the blood flows out through the stenotic valve opening. This is analogous to the flow of a stream which is silent until it is accelerated by passage between rocks.

A systolic murmur can also be caused by leakage of the tricuspid valve or the mitral valve and in this case the murmur is due to part of the blood being squirted backwards in a noisy jet into the atrium.

Diastolic murmurs can also occur between contractions when the heart is filling. These murmurs can originate either from blood leaking back through the pulmonic or aortic valves or from an obstruction to filling through a narrowed mitral or tricuspid valve.

Murmurs can also occur in patients with certain types of congenital heart defects. Sometimes these murmurs are due to congenital malformations of one or more of the heart valves, or to the persistence of an embryonic defect in the atrial or ventricular septum.

So in dealing with a heart murmur the main question is not whether or not a murmur is present, but rather what is causing it. A thorough investigation can determine the cause of the murmur and allow for the separation of those who need treatment from those who do not.

While it is possible for any of the four heart valves to be the cause of a murmur, it is usually the aortic and/or the mitral valve which are responsible.

When rheumatic fever was common, it was the most frequent cause of damage to the heart valves. The valves usually affected were the mitral and aortic valves, and until recently, rheumatic heart disease was the most common reason for aortic or mitral valve replacement. Fortunately, rheumatic fever is now very rare; and it is unusual, even in a busy cardiology practice, to see a patient with this condition.

Now the most common cause of aortic valve disease is congenital malformation. The aortic valve has three leaflets which if developed normally are of equal size. Occasionally, however, during the development of the aortic valve these leaflets do not form properly, and two of the three leaflets remain fused resulting in a bicuspid rather that the usual tricuspid valve structure.

This abnormally formed valve is out of balance and because of this imbalance, with the millions of openings and closings it undergoes, it wears out more quickly than a normal valve, much like a car tire that is out of balance. In an attempt to repair this valve the body lays down fibrous tissue on the valve — a sort-of biologic Bondo — which over time thickens and stiffens the valve preventing it from closing properly. This faulty closure causes the valve to leak (aortic regurgitation or insufficiency) and the resultant leak can be heard as a murmur during the relaxation phase (or diastole). As the fibrous repair job turns to scar tissue and shrinks, the opening of the aortic valve is narrowed, obstructing the normal flow of blood out of the heart (aortic stenosis). The turbulent jet of blood passing through the narrowed valve produces a murmur which can be heard during contraction of the heart (or systole)

When this leak or obstruction becomes severe, the heart cannot continue to force the blood through the tiny hole, the heart becomes overloaded and congestive heart failure develops. If the heart failure cannot be controlled medically, surgical replacement of the valve is required.

> *If it weren't for the surgery, I wouldn't be here today.*
> Bundy — Age 60. Heart valve disease

With the disappearance of rheumatic heart disease, the most common cause of mitral valve dysfunction is not damage to the valve itself, but to the heart muscle to which the valve is attached.

The two mitral valve leaflets are hinged along the sides and the free edges are tethered down to the inside of the left ventricle by parachute-like shrouds that prevent the valve leaflets from blowing back into the atrium when the heart contracts. If the heart muscle to which the valve leaflets are anchored is damaged, these tethers become lax, and the valve does not close properly allowing blood to leak backward during ventricular contraction. This leak can be heard as a murmur in systole. If this leakage becomes severe the heart can become overloaded, and heart failure can develop. As with aortic valve disease, medical treatment, described in Chapter 8, is often effective in controlling the heart failure; but if not, mitral valve replacement is required.

Prior to recommending valve replacement, the cardiologist and the surgeon will want to confirm the need for surgery by performing a cardiac catheterization. In this procedure small tubes or catheters are inserted into an artery and a vein, usually in the leg, and floated back up to the heart with the guidance of a fluoroscope. When the tip of the catheters are in place, the pressure on both sides of the heart can be measured and the amount of valve damage can be confirmed. As part of the procedure, pictures are made of the coronary arteries so that coronary artery by-pass can be done at the time of the valve replacement, if necessary. The catheterization procedure is done in an x-ray room, not an operating room, no surgery is performed and no general anaesthesia required. Patients remain awake during the procedure and can go home later in the same day.

There are a variety of mechanical heart valves which have been developed over the past thirty-five years. More recently, biologic or tissue valves salvaged from pigs or from human cadavers have become available. Both mechanical and tissue valves are effective. The choice of which to use is usually made by the surgeon after discussing the pros and cons of each with the patient. Each valve has its advantages and disadvantages, and most surgeons feel that no one valve is preferable in all circumstances.

One disadvantage of mechanical valves which has not yet been overcome is their tendency to get sticky with small blood clots. These clots can interfere with the valve function, causing it to stick open or closed. Pieces of blood clot can become dislodged and be swept away by the circulation to damage the brain or other vital organs. To prevent this anticoagulants are routinely prescribed for patients with mechanical heart valves. The most commonly prescribed anticoagulant is Coumadin which is the brand name for bis-hydroxy coumadin, a naturally occurring compound first discovered in moldy clover hay. As is often the case in medical science, this was discovered by chance when a herd of dairy cattle in Wisconsin got into some moldy clover hay and died as a result of massive internal hemorrhage.

After an intensive investigation the active ingredient was isolated and it has been in clinical use for the past thirty years. Taking Coumadin is not without risk. Coumadin is also the active ingredient in the rat poison Decon, which kills rats like it killed the cows. However with regular monitoring of blood tests, the risk of taking this drug has been minimized and for patients with mechanical heart valves is considerably less than the risk of not taking it.

It is important to emphasize that patients taking Coumadin cannot take aspirin, or medicines containing aspirin since this can potentiate the anticoagulant effects of Coumadin and greatly increase the risk of hemorrhage.

CHAPTER 6

MITRAL VALVE PROLAPSE

What Is Mitral Valve Prolapse Anyway?

By far, the worst thing about mitral valve prolapse is the name. It has a sinister ring to it, like muscular dystrophy or osteomyelitis. However, for the most part, mitral valve prolapse is a medical curiosity and in talking with patients who have it, I spend most of my time reassuring them that this terrible sounding thing that has attracted so much attention is not likely to either change their life or shorten it.

The story of mitral valve prolapse began when doctors noticed that some healthy, young patients had an extra heart sound or "click". In addition to the usual "LUB-DUP" that the normal heart makes, these patients hearts went "LUB-*CLICK*-DUP". The origin of this extra sound remained a mystery until the development of the echocardiogram.

In the early 1950s, a Swedish naval radar technician proposed using sonar to study the human heart, reasoning that if sonar can "see" a ship through the fog, it might be able to "see" the structures within the heart. Using this technique he discovered, as he suspected, that the movements of the heart and heart valves could be clearly visualized, and for the first time the origin of the mysterious extra click was demonstrated.

The leaflets of the mitral valve are hinged to the heart wall and their free edge is tethered down by cord-like structures to keep it from inverting back into the atrium when it is closed by ventricular contraction. Ordinarily the two leaflets of the mitral valve close together flat, like the doors of a double gate, reopening when the ventricle relaxes to fill. (Figure 1, see page 2)

In patients with mitral valve prolapse, one of the mitral valve leaflets is larger than it needs to be and when this valves closes, part of it may protrude — or prolapse — backwards slightly into the atrium. This prolapse can be seen on echocardiography, and the instant this prolapse is arrested by the tensed chords coincides exactly with the click which can be heard with the stethoscope.

So the problem, if there is one, in patients with mitral valve prolapse is that their mitral valve is larger than it needs to be. But it's like having big feet or big ears. They work perfectly well. The large mitral valve leaflet just makes a funny noise.

Mitral valve prolapse is quite common, especially, for some reason in slender women. I see two or three patients with mitral valve prolapse in my practice each week. It is said to occur in some form in about ten percent of the population, which would be the same frequency as diabetes. It is also quite fashionable. You can hardly pick up a health magazine or a women's magazine these days without seeing something on mitral valve prolapse. When I look out into the reception room and see among the older patients a thin, young woman waiting to see me, I can be relatively certain that she has mitral valve prolapse.

Most patients with mitral valve prolapse don't know they have it till they are told so by some well-meaning physician who hears the characteristic click at the time of a routine physical examination. Most have no symptoms whatsoever, and many may never have any. Some patients with mitral valve prolapse have chest pains, palpitations or tachycardia; but since all patients with mitral valve prolapse do not have symptoms and since these same symptoms can occur in patients without mitral valve prolapse, it is difficult to know whether or not the prolapse has anything to do with the symptoms.

The magazines which feature discussions of mitral valve prolapse point out dire consequences which are said to be attributed to this condition. Patients with mitral valve prolapse are said to be prone to strokes and sudden death; but instances of this must be exceptionally rare. I do not recall one such occurrence in thirty years.

No specific treatment is required for mitral valve prolapse. Those patients with tachycardia may require some treatment to control the tachycardia, as those without mitral valve prolapse might. The chest pain is usually of little consequence except when it confuses physicians into believing that it may be due to coronary artery disease. Fortunately most of the patients with mitral valve prolapse are young, well below the coronary age group. If necessary, a treadmill test or a isotope scan can settle the issue. Occasionally a coronary angiogram is required to exclude coronary artery disease completely, especially in older patients.

In some patients with mitral valve prolapse, the prolapsing valve leaks slightly. The turbulence from this leak can roughen up the surface of the valve leaflet. This roughening can, in rare instances, predispose to infection on the valve, a condition known as bacterial endocarditis. Although this is quite rare, it can be life threatening if it occurs. Because of this possibility, the American Heart Association recommends that patients whose valve leaks take an antibiotic at the time of dental work, a procedure which regularly introduces bacteria into the blood stream for a brief period. Most dentists are well aware of this recommendation. Antibiotics are not recommended for ordinary skin infection or sterile surgery, but are recommended for vaginal childbirth or surgical procedures on the bladder, nose, mouth or bowel.

It is important to emphasize that this antibiotic precaution is just that — a precaution — and that the chances of developing an infection on one of these valves is exceedingly small. This recommendation is another example of physicians erring on the side of caution and should in no way undermine the reassurance about mitral valve prolapse in general.

Patients with mitral valve prolapse should be encouraged to lead as normal a life as possible without any specific limitations or restrictions. It is conventional to recommend that patients with mitral valve prolapse have check-ups, perhaps every two to five years, primarily for the reassurance of both the patient and the physician that all continues to go well.

Echocardiograms are sometimes used to supplement the regular exam as a way of monitoring the amount of valve leakage if it is present.

The fact that the valve leaks is generally of no consequence. The issue is how much it leaks. Occasionally the amount of leakage increases with time, and this can be detected with an echocardiogram.

If the leakage increases to the point that the heart is under some strain medical treatment or, in very unusual circumstances, valve replacement may be required. But the percentage of patients with mitral valve prolapse ever requiring any treatment is exceedingly small.

Patients are often upset when they are first told that they have mitral valve prolapse, but the passage of time and the absence of symptoms continue to reinforce the idea that for most patients, mitral valve prolapse is little more than a variation of normal

CHAPTER 7

HYPERTENSION
High Blood Pressure: The Silent Killer

High blood pressure (or hypertension) is probably the most prevalent abnormality of the cardiovascular system. According to the American Heart Association, 50 million Americans have high blood pressure, and most are not even aware of it.

While there are several known causes of hypertension (such as disorders of the kidney and adrenal glands), in most cases the exact cause of a patient's high blood pressure is not known; and it is labeled, for lack of a better term, "essential hypertension."

Hypertension is most common in older patients, but it can develop in younger patients as well. Often, in the beginning, the blood pressure is labile, that is, the blood pressure fluctuates from hour to hour and from day to day depending on factors which are not well understood. Sometimes the pressure is elevated and sometimes it is not. This variation can lead the patient and the physician to assume that there may be no problem. But it is important to recognize that for the blood pressure to EVER be elevated is abnormal, and that this phase of labile hypertension should initiate concern and closer observation rather than complacency. Eventually labile hypertension becomes "fixed" and the blood pressure is then elevated on all occasions.

So called "white coat hypertension" is a myth that does not serve the patient well. This term is sometimes used to refer to patients who only have high blood pressure at the doctor's office. I was often told by patients, "Gee, Doc, my blood pressure is only elevated when I come to see you."

While this may seem true, it is usually not; and this attitude is only a form of denial or misunderstanding. Patients with high blood pressure are simply those who respond to the stresses of life by raising their blood pressure. If all it takes to raise it is a trip to the doctor, it is likely that traffic jams or family problems will do the same.

Patients respond to life's stresses in different ways. Some by getting headaches. Some by getting ulcers. Some by getting diarrhea. And some by raising their blood pressure. Usually patients who respond physically to stress do so in the same way each time, but each of these responses to stress is abnormal.

Recognizing these patterns and attempting to deal with the stress is sometimes helpful, but often the tendency to develop high blood pressure in response to stress is unavoidable.

The danger, of course, is that over a period of years, the high blood pressure damages the blood vessels, strains the heart and can lead to stroke, kidney damage and heart failure.

Most patients are not aware that they have high blood pressure, and it is difficult to detect except by direct measurement. This lack of symptoms has led hypertension to be referred to as "the silent killer."

With each heart beat the pressure generated by the heart pump is transmitted to the arteries to circulate the blood. The highest pressure generated is called the "systolic" pressure — the top number of the blood pressure reading, i.e., the 120 of the 120 over 80. As the heart relaxes, the blood pressure falls until the aortic valve closes, preventing any further drop, and this lowest pressure is called the "diastolic" pressure — the bottom number of the reading.

The blood pressure is measured with the familiar blood pressure cuff, or sphygmomanometer. The cuff is applied to the upper arm and inflated above the expected systolic blood pressure level. This temporarily stops blood flow to the arm. While listening with a stethoscope over the artery below the cuff, the pressure in the cuff is slowly released. When the pressure in the cuff is just exceeded by the pressure in the artery, blood flow is resumed and a pulsing sound can be heard through the stethoscope. The pressure indicated on the gauge at this point is recorded as the systolic pressure. As the pressure in the blood pressure cuff is released further, the pulsing sound stops, and this number is recorded as the diastolic pressure.

High diastolic blood pressure is thought to be more serious than high systolic pressure; but systolic hypertension, which is more common in the elderly, is also dangerous and requires treatment.

The goal in treating hypertension is to normalize the blood pressure under all circumstances without producing unacceptable side effects. Prior to the availability of effective blood pressure lowering agents, sedatives and tranquilizers were used in an attempt to blunt the patient's response to stress. The blood pressure control provided by these drugs was inconsistent, and the side effects were often disabling. Presently, the drugs available for the control of hypertension are numerous, safe and effective. Most of these drugs are vasodilators of some sort.

The underlying problem in patients with hypertension is that, for some reason, the blood vessels in the body are constricted. As a consequence the pressure in the entire arterial system is elevated. It is as if there is too much circulating adrenalin constantly readying the patient for "fight or flight." Perhaps, for some reason, they secrete too much adrenalin; or perhaps they are just excessively sensitive to it. Many medical conditions which we consider abnormal are, in fact, just excessive variations of normal.

Vasodilators relax these constricted vessels and allow the blood pressure to return toward normal. The dose of the vasodilator is critical. Too much and the blood pressure drops too low. Too little and the blood pressure is uncontrolled.

The treatment of hypertension with vasodilators usually requires some period of time to adjust the medication to the proper dose. Each patient is different. It is, like many other things in medicine, a matter of educated trial and error. It is hard to predict in advance what the best dose, or even the best drug will be.

Many drug choices are now available for the treatment of hypertension, and it is possible to control the blood pressure in virtually all patients using one or a combination of these agents. In addition to vasodilators, one of the stand-bys of hypertension treatment is diuretics, or so called "water pills." For some reason patients with high blood pressure avidly retain sodium, even the small amount that they may eat on a salt-restricted diet. Sodium contributes to the increased vascular constriction which further raises the intra-arterial pressure. Diuretics block the avid salt retention by the kidney and allow it to be excreted. Water is excreted along with the sodium hence the name, "water pills."

Some of the stronger diuretics cause loss of potassium in addition to sodium. Potassium is very difficult to replace in the normal diet, even by increasing the intake of potassium containing foods such as citrus fruit and bananas. It is not uncommon for a patient taking diuretics to lose forty to sixty units of potassium a day, and a glass of orange juice or a banana each contain only eight units. Patients taking diuretics often require potassium supplements. Many salt substitutes contain potassium chloride rather than sodium chloride, and these products may be a valuable source of additional dietary potassium.

Another class of drugs used for the control of hypertension is the beta blockers. These drugs block the so-called beta receptor, the receptor in the arterial wall for compounds like adrenalin which can cause increased vascular constriction. With these receptor sites blocked by a beta blocker drug, the effect of circulating adrenalin-like compounds is decreased and vascular constriction decreases.

It is important to realize that high blood pressure can never be cured — only controlled. Once a patient has identified himself as hypertensive, medical treatment of some type is required for life. If the medicine controlling the blood pressure is stopped, the blood pressure will simply return to the previously elevated level. It is as if the pressure in that patient is just set higher.

It is also important to emphasize that if the blood pressure is controlled, the patient should be able to live a perfectly healthy and long life. Hypertension does no other damage except by virtue of the elevated blood pressure. So when the blood pressure is controlled, the risk is removed.

Prior to using any medication it is important that the patient reduce their weight to their ideal body weight. Some patients with hypertension are not overweight, but many are and if so, it is important to reduce the excess body weight. Sometimes this is not possible, but nonetheless it is the first line of treatment. Many patients who are overweight find that they can reduce, or even eliminate, their blood pressure medicine once their weight has returned to normal.

A restriction of sodium intake is also critical. Most of the sodium patients receive is in the form of dietary salt or sodium chloride. It is not possible to completely eliminate sodium from the diet, and it is useless to try to do so. However, the dietary salt intake can easily be reduced by paying attention to the diet. This requires that patients understand where dietary sodium comes from.

By now everyone understands that they should restrict the use of salt at the table by eliminating it altogether or by using a salt substitute. Those who find this diet unpalatable sometimes get satisfaction using vinegar or lemon juice (which mimics the sour taste of the chloride in the sodium chloride) or by using one of several available spice combinations. Salt cooked in the food counts the same as salt added to the food after it is cooked. Cooking the salt provides no protection.

In addition to restricting the use of salt at the table or in cooking, patients need to realize that many foods already contain salt. Foods which contain the highest amounts of salt are prepared foods such as frozen dinners, prepared meats, and snack foods such as pickles, olives, peanut butter and chips. One package of potato chips contains about one third of the salt that a person on a salt-restricted diet should take during the entire day.

Perhaps the most deceptive food, and one which fools the most patients, is soup — either dried or canned. In my experience this is one of the most common sources of salt in the diets of those patients who are trying to restrict it. Often these patients are on weight reduction diets or are older patients, and soup is an easily prepared, low calorie meal. However the amount of salt in soup is very high, and patients on salt restricted diets should either avoid soup entirely, restrict it as much as possible, or better yet, eat homemade soup made with a salt substitute.

Nicotine can raise the blood pressure and patients with high blood pressure should quit using it. The popularity of snuff among young people is particularly worrisome since it not only contains nicotine but also a large amount of salt. Thus it is not much help, if blood pressure control is the goal, to switch from cigarettes to snuf. The same can be said for nicotine patches which can produce high blood pressure; and, in my experience, sometimes merely re-addict patients who have already almost quit smoking.

The accepted goal for hypertension treatment is a diastolic blood pressure of no higher than 80 and a systolic blood pressure of 140. Reduction of elevated blood pressure to these levels — even among the elderly — reduces the risk of complications by thirty percent!

The role of stress management and bio-feedback is likewise not well defined, but sometimes this form of treatment can be helpful, and in patients who are motivated, it is certainly worth a try.

It is important to point out that hypertension tends to run in families and it should be looked for in relatives of patients with high blood pressure. The most important thing about hypertension is to look for it and if you find it, get it fixed. With all of the resources we have at our disposal, there is simply no excuse for having high blood pressure.

CHAPTER 8

CONGESTIVE HEART FAILURE
If I Have Heart Failure, How Come I Am Still Alive?

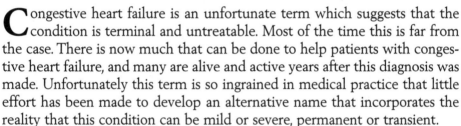

Congestive heart failure is an unfortunate term which suggests that the condition is terminal and untreatable. Most of the time this is far from the case. There is now much that can be done to help patients with congestive heart failure, and many are alive and active years after this diagnosis was made. Unfortunately this term is so ingrained in medical practice that little effort has been made to develop an alternative name that incorporates the reality that this condition can be mild or severe, permanent or transient.

Congestive heart failure develops when there is enough weakness of the heart muscle that the heart can no longer function adequately. This can be the result of permanent damage from a heart attack, or from bad valves that overload the heart, or a transient viral infection of the heart muscle. Whatever the cause, heart failure results when the heart can no longer pump blood forward fast enough to meet the body's demands. Symptoms result both from the stagnation of blood "behind" the pump and the slowed forward flow to the vital organs.

When the blood returning to the heart is not moved along, it tends to dam up in the spongy substance of the lungs. This stiffens the lungs, decreasing their normal elasticity and flexibility, creating the sensation of shortness of breath from the extra effort required to inflate the stiffened lungs. This shortness of breath is particularly noticeable on exertion or on lying down when gravity tends to congest the distended lungs even more.

When the forward blood flow to the body is reduced, this reduced flow is detected by special sensors in the kidneys which "interpret" this reduced flow as low blood volume. They "think" the blood has leaked out; and, perhaps the remnant of a survival instinct, the kidneys attempt to preserve blood volume at all costs, avidly retaining fluid. This increased fluid is exactly what the body does NOT need, and it further stresses the already weakened heart and accumulates in the lungs, where it worsens the sensation of shortness of breath and in the soft tissue where it accumulates under the influence of gravity as leg swelling or edema.

The medical treatment of congestive heart failure has developed along three lines. The traditional approach is to strengthen the heart's pumping action using digitalis, a chemical derived from the foxglove that grew in your grandmother's garden. Digitalis has been used in this way since the time of George Washington when it was discovered by a physician-botanist named William Withering to be the active ingredient in the brew of an English witch.

The second line of defense in congestive heart failure is the use of diuretics or "water pills." These agents act to selectively reduce the kidneys' efforts at salt and water retention and allow the body to rid itself of the excess fluid. An integral part of this effort to reduce body fluid is an effort to limit the dietary intake of sodium, most of which is available as sodium chloride, or salt. Most of the salt in the diet, besides that which is added at the table, comes from snack food such as pickles, crackers, olives and chips. The amount of salt in a package of potato chips is one third of the daily allotment for a person on a salt-restricted diet.

Another often unsuspected source of salt is canned and prepared foods — foods such as TV dinners and canned or dried soup — often the staples of elderly people who live alone and cook for themselves.

The third approach uses vasodilator drugs which are popularly referred to as "unloading" agents. These medicines are a group of drugs which dilate blood vessels throughout the body, lowering the blood pressure against which the heart has to work and thereby facilitating forward flow.

It has recently been discovered that beta blocker drugs can also be helpful in the treatment of congestive heart failure.

Treatment with these drugs can often have a remarkably beneficial effect on the symptoms of heart failure, and patients with severe limitations prior to treatment can often return to activity that is near-normal for their age. Sometimes the underlying cause of the heart failure can be surgically corrected, but if not, medical treatment can provide relief from the fluid retention that causes most of the symptoms.

Diseases of the heart valves, especially the aortic and mitral valves, can also interfere with the efficient pumping action of the heart and, if severe enough, can result in heart failure by overloading the heart. The medical treatment outlined above is often effective in relieving the symptoms of heart failure caused by valve disease. But in some cases the valve disease progresses to the point where medical treatment is no longer effective and surgical replacement of the diseased valve or valves is required for relief. The timing of valve replacement is critical. If done too early, the risk of surgery is not accompanied by much benefit. If too late, the heart has dilated in an attempt to accommodate to the increased workload due to the leaking or obstructed valve and is so stretched out of shape that it cannot recover even if the valve is replaced. Like a water pump, a bad valve, if ignored for too long, can burn the pump out.

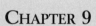

CHAPTER 9

PACEMAKERS

My Grandmother Had a Pacemaker and She Died

Cardiac pacemakers are another example of the many technological advances that have benefited patients with heart disease. Since their introduction in the late 1960s, these remarkable devices have undergone a steady series of improvements and have benefited thousands of patients who without them would have had only a 50-50 chance of living another five years.

The normal heart rhythm is initiated by a microscopic natural pacemaker in the wall of the right atrium, one of the upper heart chambers. This tiny structure known as the sinus node, discharges spontaneously at a rate of about seventy impulses a minute. The impulse of the pacemaker spreads down over the heart through a specialized conducting system to the lower heart chambers — the ventricles — stimulating them to contract in an orderly pumping sequence.

This natural pacemaker and the conducting system can wear out just as ears, eyes and hips can wear out. If this happens the discharges from the pacemaker in the atrium cannot reach the ventricle — a condition known as heart block — and the heart rate slows, sometimes to the range of thirty beats per minute. This rate is too slow for normal circulation and can result in severe weakness, shortness of breath or sometimes loss of consciousness.

Failure of the natural pacing system can be sometimes abrupt and permanent; so that once the heart rate slows, it remains slow. Pacemaker failure, however, can sometimes be intermittent like a short in a lamp cord, causing intermittent recurrent episodes of fainting punctuated by periods of normal heart rate.

In this rather common situation, the patient's natural pacemaker can suddenly blink off and then spontaneously resume normal activity. The patient, having fainted, then arrives at the hospital recovered and with a normal heart rhythm and rate. Sometimes there are clues on the EKG that the patient might be having intermittent failure of his pacing system. Often prolonged EKG monitoring is required to detect this intermittent pacemaker failure.

Failure of the natural pacemaker is very common in the older age groups, and the resulting loss of consciousness is the cause of numerous falls and injuries. There are many causes of fainting, but in the older age group episodes of fainting should be considered due to failure of the pacing system until proven otherwise. If left untreated pacemaker failure can be fatal.

The treatment for failure of the natural pacing system is quite straightforward. The damaged natural pacemaker must be replaced with an artificial one. These systems are designed to mimic the natural system and maintain a normal heart rate. If the natural pacemaker has failed completely the artificial pacemaker will operate all the time. If the failure of the natural pacemaker is intermittent, the artificial pacemaker will be activated only when it is needed, functioning like the thermostat in a home furnace. If the heart rate drops below a certain set level, the pacemaker switches on and restores the heart to normal. When the natural pacemaker begins to function again, the heart rate rises and the artificial pacemaker is shut off.

Ordinarily, the pacemaker will pace the heart at a certain pre-set rate. There are now pacemakers which can adjust their rate to a patient's activity level. In one model, the jiggling of the pacemaker caused by exercise, causes the pacemaker to increase its pacing rate.

Pacemakers are effective only for patients with slow heart rates. Pacemakers do not strengthen the heart beat nor do they control episodes of rapid heart action.

Implantation of a permanent artificial pacemaker is a minor operation and is usually quite well tolerated, even by the elderly. There is no need for general anesthesia, and the procedure is usually completed within half an hour. The skin under the collar bone is anesthetized with novocaine, a small incision is made and the pacemaker is placed under the skin. The pacemaker is connected to the heart by a small coated wire which is inserted into a vein and floated back down into the heart. The passage of this catheter through the veins to the heart is not accompanied by any unpleasant sensation. When the pacemaker and the coated wire are in the proper position, the skin is sewn up. Following the implantation of a pacemaker the patient usually leaves the hospital the next day and is encouraged to resume normal activities.

> *If I felt any better, you'd have to put a guard on me.*
> Luther — Age 78. Pacemaker patient

Early models of pacemakers were about the size of an English muffin, but have now been reduced to about the size of a pocket watch, and their shape cannot be noticed under normal clothing. Batteries which once lasted only twelve to eighteen months now routinely last ten years. When they run down, they are simply replaced.

When first developed, the circuits of the pacemaker could be affected by interference from nearby electrical fields and patients with pacemakers were advised not to use electrical appliances or hand tools or even electric razors. Engineers have now designed pacemakers so that they are not affected by this outside electrical interference, including microwave ovens. Metal detectors at the airports will, of course, detect the pacemaker but will in no way damage it or affect its function.

Although almost flawless, pacemakers are electrical gadgets. While failure is extremely rare, it does occur. Therefore routine follow-up is required. Thanks to modern technology, much of this follow-up can be done from the patient's home using a small electrical device which transmits a record of the pacemaker's function over the telephone to a special receiver. The number of visits to the doctor's office can be minimized. This is particularly helpful for older patients who have difficulty traveling. These transtelephonic pacemaker checks are part of the routine follow up of patients with pacemakers.

Depending on the type of pacemaker, patients are also seen in the office once or twice a year for a more complete pacemaker check at which time adjustments can be made if necessary. These adjustments can be made electronically through the intact skin within a matter of minutes.

Pacemakers run on batteries, and batteries can run down. If so the batteries have to be replaced. Since the batteries are sealed within the pacemaker itself, the batteries cannot be changed, and the entire pacemaker requires replacement. For this the skin over the pacemaker is anesthetized with lidocaine, a small incision is made exposing the pacemaker which is simply unscrewed from the end of the pacing catheter and replaced with a new unit in a matter of a few minutes.

It is sometimes difficult for patients who did not have electricity in the house when they were born to adjust to the idea that they are "living on a battery." They have seen batteries fail and they are concerned about blinking off like an old flashlight.

However engineers have designed modern pacemakers so that as the batteries fail, the heart rate slows gradually over a period of months. This and other electronic changes can easily be detected by pacemaker interrogation systems either over the telephone or in the doctor's office. If the batteries begin to run down, they are simply replaced.

It is possible for pacing to fail abruptly if the wire from the pacemaker to the heart breaks; but this is exceedingly rare, and often there are warning signs that can be detected during the regular pacemaker checkups.

Some patients with pacemakers also have extensive heart disease and because of that may have limitations. On the other hand many patients have no other heart trouble except that their natural pacemaker is worn out. In these patients the placement of an artificial pacemaker restores the heart to normal function for their age, and they are capable of leading normal lives. Therefore, whether a patient with a pacemaker has any limitations depends not on the presence of the pacemaker, but on the overall condition of the heart. If a pacemaker is the patient's only heart problem, physicians do not place any restrictions or limitations on his activities.

The best thing a patient with a pacemaker can do is to forget about it and let the doctor do the checking.

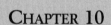

Chapter 10

CONGENITAL HEART DISEASE
If It Can Go Wrong It Will

The term congenital heart disease refers to a group of heart conditions that result from faulty development of the heart. These conditions, by definition, are always present from birth.

The development of the heart is an intricately complex process and considering the exact orchestration required, it is a wonder, not that this process occasionally fails to work perfectly, but that the heart normally works as well as it does.

Congenital heart disease is an example of a sort of biologic Murphy's Law — if it can go wrong, sooner or later it will. If there is a fault of alignment or growth or timing at any of the numerous stages of this complex process, a congenital heart defect can result.

Congenital heart defects are not random, but are predictable events — the result of failures at very specific developmental stages. Some defects are more common than others, but defects during the formation of all the heart structures are possible and do occur. Congenital heart defects can involve the heart chambers, the heart muscle, the heart valves and even the tiny heart pacemaker. Some of the more common defects are discussed below. **(Figure 4)**

In an almost irresistible inclination to simplify, medical scientists have arbitrarily divided all congenital heart defects into two major groups — those that cause cyanosis (a term used to describe the blue discoloration of the skin which results from inadequate oxygen in the blood) and those that do not.

Cyanotic heart diseases are conditions that result from defects in the heart that allow the venous blood, headed for the lungs, to mix with arterial blood headed for the body.

One example of cyanotic congenital heart disease is the so-called Tetralogy of Fallot, named for the 18th-century physician who described

FIGURE 4

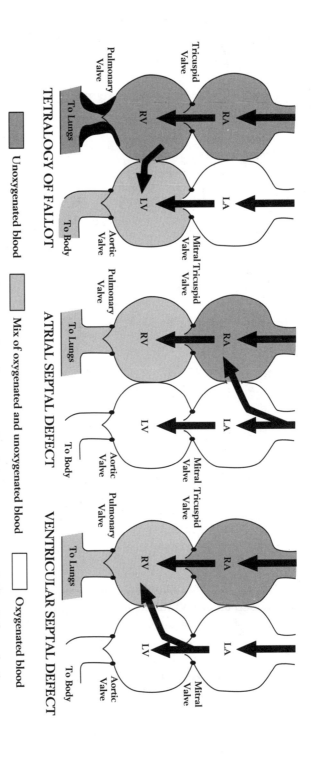

TETRALOGY OF FALLOT

Tricuspid Valve
Pulmonary Valve
To Lungs
RV
RA
LV
LA
Aortic Valve
Mitral Valve
Tricuspid Valve
To Body

ATRIAL SEPTAL DEFECT

Pulmonary Valve
To Lungs
RV
RA
LV
LA
Aortic Valve
Mitral Valve
Tricuspid Valve
To Body

VENTRICULAR SEPTAL DEFECT

Pulmonary Valve
To Lungs
RV
RA
LV
LA
Aortic Valve
Mitral Valve
To Body

■ Unoxygenated blood

▨ Mix of oxygenated and unoxygenated blood

□ Oxygenated blood

TETRALOGY OF FALLOT: The narrowed (stenotic) pulmonary valve forces unoxygenated blood from body across a defect in the ventricular septum to mix with oxygenated blood from lungs.

ATRIAL SEPTAL DEFECT: Oxygenated blood from lungs crosses a defect in the atrial septum to mix with unoxygenated blood from body.

VENTRICULAR SEPTAL DEFECT: Oxygenated blood from lungs crosses a defect in the ventricular septum to mix with unoxygenated blood from the body.

it. It is the most common cause of "blue babies." In this condition the valve from the heart to the lungs does not develop to an adequate size and remains too small to allow enough of the blood returning to the heart to pass through to the lungs. Because of this obstruction to normal blood flow, the blood is diverted from the right side of the heart, through a persistently patent defect in the septum dividing the two sides of the heart. Since this diverted venous blood by-passes the lungs, its oxygen content remains very low. When this diverted blood mixes with the oxygenated blood in the left side of the heart, the resultant mix that is pumped out to the body has a lower-than-normal oxygen content.

Most of the cyanotic congenital heart defects are a variation on this basic defect — a predictable persistence, if you will, of the situation *in utero* where the blood returning to the heart is diverted from the unused lungs. After birth, however, there is no longer a maternal placenta to supply the oxygen.

Fortunately most of these defects are now surgically correctable. The persistent defect in the ventricular septum can be sewn closed or patched, and the underdeveloped valve can be enlarged or replaced allowing a normal flow to the lungs.

> *Before I was treated, I was so sick and depressed I*
> *wanted to kill myself. Now I have gone back to coaching*
> *field hockey.*
> Jeanette — Age 27 Congenital heart disease patient

The most common of the non-cyanotic congenital heart defects is the atrial septal defect which is due to the failure of the hole between the right and left atriums to close at birth. Since the pressure in the left side of the heart is greater than the right, some of the blood returning from the lungs is diverted across this atrial defect and back into the lungs. A similar situation exists if the hole between the left and right ventricles does not close. This is referred to as a ventricular septal defect. If either of these persistent holes is large enough, it must be surgically closed to prevent the extra blood flow from damaging the lungs.

You can imagine the dismay that youngsters must feel when they are told, as it is sometimes put, that they have a hole in their heart. How unfortunate some of our terminology is. I always make a special effort when talking with these children to make sure that they understand that they do not have a hole in their heart which no one else has, but that one of the holes which everyone has in their hearts has simply not yet closed.

The most common congenital valve defect affects the aortic valve, the valve between the left ventricle and the aorta. This check valve is designed to prevent blood which has been pumped from the heart from flowing back into it. Normally this valve has three leaflets, each of equal size. In some patients, however, the leaflets do not divide properly, and two remain fused together. This deformed valve does not close properly, and blood can leak back into the heart after each contraction. If the leak is large enough, the additional blood volume can eventually overload the heart.

In addition, since the valve is out of balance, it wears out faster than normal, much like an automobile tire out of balance. The body attempts to repair the worn valve by laying down scar tissue, but in time this scar tissue shrinks and stiffens the valve to the point that it can neither open nor close properly and it must be replaced.

Most children with non-cyanotic congenital heart defects can and should lead normal active lives with the possible exception of competitive sports which need to be restricted for those with more severe defects. Surgery, if required, is usually deferred until the teenage years when the defect can almost always be completely corrected, nowadays at very low risk. It is worth whatever effort is required to remind these children that they are not really so different from normal; and that after surgical correction their hearts will be as good as yours and mine and their lives just as long.

CHAPTER 11

LESS COMMON HEART CONDITIONS:
Infections, Heart Muscle Disease and Pericarditis

〜

One of the most dreaded of all heart conditions is infection on the heart valves. This is known as infective endocarditis or, since almost all infections on heart valves are bacterial in origin, bacterial endocarditis.

In this condition, bacteria infect the heart valves themselves, usually just one valve, but occasionally two. These infections almost invariably occur on heart valves previously damaged (usually by rheumatic fever) though any damaged valve, including congenitally deformed valves, are vulnerable to infection. It is important to note that the normal heart valve is very resistant to infection

One of the dangers of infective endocarditis is that it is an indolent disease which begins very slowly and is often not manifest by distinctive symptoms until late in the disease when treatment is exceedingly difficult. The infection grows slowly, destroying or dissolving the heart valve and making it leak which puts an extra work load on the heart. In addition, bits of infection on the heart valve can be blown away by the force of the blood stream spreading the infection to all parts of the body. Larger pieces of the infected material can be swept up to the brain where they can occlude a blood vessel causing a stroke. Sometimes the infection spreads to the brain as a result of this seeding, causing abcesses in the brain tissue.

The symptoms of infective endocarditis are often very non-specific and include low grade fever (which is often not noticed) a change in the sound of a previously detected heart murmur (indicating more damage to the valves) and sometimes, in the terminal phases, weight loss.

Unfortunately too often the first sign of bacterial endocarditis is a stroke. Stroke in a young person should always raise the possibility of endocarditis, particularly if the patient has a preexisting valve condition.

Infection of a heart valve is thought to result from bacteria which get into the circulation through a break in the skin or an infection elsewhere in the body. One of the frequent sources is a dental infection from which bacteria enter the blood stream and set up an infection on one of the heart valves.

The treatment of bacterial endocarditis involves the use of intravenous antibiotics in large doses requiring hospitalization for up to six weeks. The infection is very difficult to eradicate, and long-term treatment is required.

Since the consequences of endocarditis are so grave, great effort has been made to prevent this infection in susceptible individuals. It is recommended that patients with damaged heart valves take antibiotics at the time of dental work and certain types of surgery in order to prevent this terrible infection.

Bacteria can be detected in the blood stream of almost everyone in the first few hours following dental work. The bacteria are usually cleared promptly from the blood stream and do not affect normal heart valves; but if the heart valve is damaged, an infection can take place. Antibiotics given at the time of dental work can prevent these infections.

It is important to emphasize that the chance of infection, even on an abnormal valve after dental work, is very small; but since the consequences can be disastrous, the administration of antibiotics for these patients is routine. Most dentists are well aware of this, but it is prudent for patients with heart valve abnormalities to discuss this with their physician and their dentist. Bacteria invade the blood stream after routine cleaning of the teeth as well as extensive dental surgery. Antibiotics are not recommended after routine fillings.

The pericardium is a thin fibrous bag that covers the entire heart like a sock. The most common disease of the pericardium is infection, usually by a virus. In the old days the pericardium was sometimes infected with tuberculosis, but this is very rare now. The virus infection causes inflamation of the pericardium, and the cardinal feature of this is chest pain which is sometimes confused with the pain due to heart attack. But the characteristic pain of pericarditis is pleurisy (or pain on deep breathing) usually more marked when lying down, and patients often seek comfort sitting and leaning over the back of a chair. Classically the pain on deep breathing radiates from the center of the chest up into the neck. The rubbing together of the inflamed, roughened pericardial surfaces makes a noise with every heart beat. This sound can be heard with the stethoscope and has always sounded to me like the squeak of new boots in the snow or the leathery squeak produced by rubbing two newly shined shoes together. This sound is referred to as a pericardial friction rub.

Although not always typical, when all of the characteristic features are present — that is, pleurisy and a friction rub — the diagnosis is very straight-forward. There is no specific treatment for viral pericarditis. Anti-inflamatory agents are used to relieve the discomfort. The course of the illness is usually self-limited, like the flu, lasting several days and is not associated with any long-term complications. Echocardiograms can confirm the presence of fluid in the pericardium and also can help to rule out other rare causes of pericarditis such as metastatic tumors.

Myocardium is the term used for heart muscle. Diseases of the myocardium are unusual. Perhaps the most common form is hypertrophic cardiomyopathy which is a congenital disease in which the heart muscle cells are weakened. In an effort to maintain normal function, the heart muscles grow, excessively thickening the heart and making it muscle-bound. In the early stages there are no symptoms, but later heart failure can result. This thickening of the heart muscle when it is well developed is apparent by changes on a routine electrocardiogram and can be clearly demonstrated by echocardiography.

A variety of treatments are available, usually medical, although occasionally surgery is required to remove parts of the thickened heart muscle wall which actually protrude into the cavity of the heart and interfere with blood flow.

Another form of heart muscle disease is dilated (or congestive) cardiomyopathy. This can result from any damage to the heart muscle if it is extensive enough. Perhaps the most common cause is alcoholism, but this sort of heart muscle weakening can take place as the result of viral infections (myocarditis), or other toxins such as cocaine. The specific cause is often never known.

There are no specific symptoms early in the course of the disease. The heart dilates to try to accommodate the heart muscle weakness. Once the dilitation has reached its limit, the symptoms and signs of heart failure become apparent. Medical treatment for this is sometimes effective. The offending toxin such as alcohol or cocaine must be avoided, and sometimes recovery is dramatic. Vasodilators reduce the work load of the heart allowing it to rest and recover its normal shape and function. The EKG is usually markedly abnormal, and the findings on echocardiography are characteristic showing a dilated, poorly contractile heart.

Acute myocarditis is usually caused by a virus and begins as a non-specific febrile illness like the flu. If the viral infection is severe enough the heart muscle can be weakened, and heart failure can develop. Ordinarily this is a self-limiting illness that responds to supportive measures within a few days. In some patients, however, acute myocarditis can so damage the heart that chronic congestive cardiomyopathy is the result.

CHAPTER 12

DIAGNOSIS OF HEART DISEASE
Why So Many Tests
~

I t is up to the physician to explain why a recommended test is necessary, what is to be learned from it, and how that information can be helpful in making a decision about your treatment. A certain amount of trust is required. A conscientious physician is always going to come down of the side of getting more information. Tests satisfy a need to confirm the physician's judgment. The more information he has about your condition, the more likely he is to give you the best advice.

In the old days physicians did a lot of guess work and were pretty good at it, but if a doctor guesses wrong, you lose. In dealing with something as serious as heart disease, there is simply no room for guess work. So be patient with your doctors when they recommend tests. They are only trying to be conscientious. But satisfy yourself by making sure that they explain what the test requires, what risks are involved, and how they expect to make use of the results.

In general there are two basic types of tests — invasive and non-invasive. Invasive tests are so named because performance of the test requires entering the circulation through a blood vessel with a catheter (or tube) to measure pressures in the heart or to inject x-ray contrast material to make pictures of heart structures. Invasive tests are by far the most accurate, but they are also the most expensive, the most troublesome, and there is usually some risk involved.

The most common invasive test in cardiology is cardiac catheterization. In this procedure a catheter is introduced into an artery or vein and is threaded back up to the heart using flouroscopic guidance. It sounds painful; but, in fact, there is very little discomfort involved. Local anesthesia is used at the site where the needle is introduced into the skin, and sometimes a small dose of tranquilizer is used to allay some of the patient's anxiety; but additional anesthesia is not required since there is little or no sensation as the catheter passes through the blood vessels.

Cardiac catheterizations are performed in special x-ray rooms called catheterization laboratories, which are usually in hospitals. More and more catheterizations are being done in outpatient facilities. The tests take a hour or so, depending on what is being done, and patients are routinely sent home and back to usual activities within a few hours.

Once the catheter has been placed within the circulation, a variety of tests can be performed, depending on the nature of the problem being studied. Pressures can be recorded from the heart chambers to evaluate heart function. Contrast material can be injected into the heart chambers and moving pictures made to evaluate any valve leakage and the pumping function of the heart itself. Abnormal communications between the two sides of the heart, common in congenital heart disease, can be demonstrated and their severity estimated. Dye injected into the coronary arteries can demonstrate the presence and extent of any blockages.

These are not new tests. Cardiac catheterizations have been performed for forty years and coronary angiography since 1965. Once limited to university medical centers, cardiac catheterizations are now routinely performed at community hospitals all over the country. Each year hundreds of thousands patients who have, or are suspected of having heart disease, undergo these valuable examinations.

There is a long list of terrible things that can happen during a cardiac catheterization including heart attack, stroke, damage to a blood vessel, bleeding, allergic reactions to the contrast material, and, rarely, even death. The chance of one of these complications occurring is very small. The few complications that do occur are usually in those patients in whom you would expect it — the elderly and those with severe cardiovascular and lung disease.

So as with any other procedure in medicine, the relative risks and benefits have to be weighed carefully. Is it safer to take the risk of the procedure to find out exactly what the trouble is and take care of it properly, or is it safer to take the risk of leaving it alone. It's not that one way is safe and the other is dangerous. Their are risks either way.

Since there are some risks associated with invasive testing, a number of non-invasive tests have been developed to try to avoid the risks, expense and inconvenience of cardiac catheterization. Here we have a remarkable *tour de force* of medical science and engineering. Working together over the past several years, medical scientists have developed techniques to investigate the heart that are little short of astounding in their complexity and accuracy, and in some instances, they have replaced invasive tests altogether. This is especialy true with echocardiography which has essentially eliminated the need for cardiac catheterization in sick newborn infants.

Echocardiography is essentially radar, or sonar applied to the study of the heart. High frequency sound waves are beamed through the chest wall at the heart. There is no sensation associated with these exams. The sound waves bounce off the heart structures and are displayed in "real time" motion much the way a ship can be "seen" in the fog. Echocardiography or ultrasound is used to display the heart anatomy — the valves, the heart chambers — and its function. It does not provide any direct information about the coronary arteries or the circulation to the heart itself. For this, a perfusion scan is required.

Perfusion scans employ radioisotopes which go where oxygen goes. By tagging the blood with an isotope such as thallium or technetium, it is possible to tell if the isotope (and oxygen) are getting to all parts of the heart muscle.

The usual procedure involves exercise to increase the heart's demand for oxygen. At peak exercise the isotope is injected into the blood stream and is taken up by the heart muscle. The isotopes give off energy which can be detected by special x-ray cameras.

Normally the isotope (and oxygen) are evenly distributed throughout the heart muscle so that the resulting photograph looks like a uniform white smudge. If there is disease in one or more of the coronary arteries, the flow of blood (and therefore the isotope) to that segment is limited, and the resulting image looks like a pie with a piece cut out of it, or a PAC MAN.

The perfusion scan can not only identify whether or not coronary arteries are diseased, but it can also distinguish between heart muscle which is dead from complete lack of blood supply (a heart attack), and heart muscle that is jeopardized by blood flow which is marginal. The marginal blood flow is due to partial blockage of a blood vessel which in time may become complete, cutting off blood flow to part of the heart entirely and causing a heart attack which may be fatal.

If the isotope scan immediately after exercise shows a defect in the scan image (a missing piece) it can indicate either permanently dead heart muscle or jeopardized muscle. To distinguish between these two possibilities, the scan is repeated in three to four hours. If the heart muscle is jeopardized from partial blockage of a blood vessel, three hours will allow enough time for blood to trickle by the narrowing and the resultant heart image will be whole again. If the blood vessel is completely blocked the heart muscle will be dead and the defect will persist even after four hours.

So the test to be performed depends on the question you are asking. If you want to know the function of the heart valves, the best non-invasive test is an echocardiogram. If you need to know the status of the coronary arteries, the simplest test is an exercise test. If you need a more accurate assessment of the coronary arteries, then one of the perfusion scans such as the thallium scan is used. If you want a non-invasive assessment of the overall heart function, the best test would be a radionucleide ventriculogram.

This type of ventriculogram is a heart scan, like the thallium scan, except that the nuclear isotope stays within the circulation instead of being absorbed by the heart muscle. The isotope "stains" the blood itself, if you will. Since the heart is filled with blood, a scan of the heart after an injection of the isotope shows the blood flowing through the heart and how strong the contractions of the heart are.

However none of these non-invasive tests is as accurate as a cardiac catheterization. Sometimes they are adequate, but if you do not get the information you need from a non-invasive test and important questions still remain, you need to go further. Whether or not you proceed to a cardiac catheterization depends on the nature of the questions, whether or not the information will clarify the diagnosis, how the information will effect the management of your condition and whether or not you understand the plan well enough to evaluate the relative risks.

Ordinarily catheterization will not be recommended unless the risk of the catheterization is less than leaving the suspected condition untreated. Sometimes catheterizations are done to exclude heart trouble, if that is the degree of accuracy required to ease the patient's mind. There is nothing more reassuring than to be told that your cardiac catheterization is completely normal. This essentially excludes the largest killer of Americans, and if the patient is 50 years old, nearly excludes the possibility of developing heart attack. Years are required to develop coronary artery disease, and if you don't have some sign of it by age fifty, you don't have time left to get it. Something else is going to have to get you.

Since coronary artery disease is the biggest killer, it would make sense to screen for it. If it were not for the expense and the small risk, you could build a case for doing a cardiac catheterization on everyone, say, over the age of forty to forty-five. Finding coronary artery disease would be much more effective from a public health point of view than screening for cancer of the colon by rectal exam and doing tests for blood in the stool. Cancer of the colon kills a fraction of the people that coronary disease kills. But the tests for colon cancer are cheap, so we do them.

For now we screen for coronary artery disease with stress tests. It is relatively expensive, as tests go, but the risk is negligible. A negative stress test at middle age means that there is little likelihood of a heart attack within the next five years. Without a catheterization, that's about the best we can do now. One of these days they will discover a non-invasive way to visualize the coronary arteries. Some of these techniques are already on the drawing board. When that time comes, screening for coronary disease will become as routine as a breast exam. I have great confidence that these techniques will be developed. I have great confidence in engineers when they have set their sights on a problem they want to solve. If engineers can hit the moon with a "basketball" they can find a non-invasive way to visualize the coronary arteries.

What test is done depends on the question being asked. The standard EKG is not a very good predictor of the future. It's more of an historical record. From looking at the EKG you can tell what has happened to the patient prior to the time the EKG was done — for instance whether or not the patient has had any previous heart attacks, but it is not a very good indicator of whether or not a heart attack is likely. For this, some sort of stress test is more effective. The rationale is similar to taking your car out on the interstate and running up the RPMs to see if the motor runs well at high speed. This is more likely to show up any weakness than just running it at idle.

To accurately diagnose a patient's abnormal heart rhythm, you have to "catch them at it." Since heart rhythm abnormalities are often intermittent and transient, the chance of detecting the abnormal rhythm on an ordinary EKG is small. Asking the patient to come in for an EKG when the rhythm disturbance is present is sometimes helpful, but often the heart rhythm has returned to normal before a recording can be made. Sometimes hospitalization and continuous EKG monitoring are required. This is very expensive and provides no guarantee, but it is preferable if the suspected rhythm disturbance is thought to be dangerous, such as ventricular tachycardia. In the hospital, the patient can be protected while the investigation continues.

If the rhythm disturbance is not thought to be dangerous, an ambulatory EKG recorder (Holter recorder) can be used to record the patient's heart rhythm while they go about their everyday duties. Since the recordings last only twenty-four hours, this too, is a random sample. There are recorders which the patient can activate when symptoms develop, and these units increase the odds of detecting intermittent heart rhythm abnormalities.

These recording devices are an example of the cross-cultural exchange between scientific disciplines. The electrodes by which the recorder is connected to the patient were developed by the space program for long-term monitoring of astronauts. Without these electrodes, long-term patient monitoring would not be possible.

So, the choice of tests depends on the question which needs to be answered and the urgency of getting the answer. It is important for the physician and the patient to discuss the tests planned, the rationale for the test, what the test is expected to show, and how this information will be useful in the patient's management. In my experience patients are very seldom resistant to "tests" if they have the opportunity to participate in this kind of discussion.

CHAPTER 13

TREATMENT OF HEART DISEASE
Can It Be Fixed?

Medical science has made progress that borders on the near-miraculous since the turn of the century when a patient was as likely as not to benefit from contact with a physician. Nowhere has this progress been more remarkable than in the treatment of heart disease.

Consider the advances in cardiac surgery. The first surgical correction of a congenital heart defect was performed in 1940. In 1961, a medical school classmate of mine who went for consultation at a major medical center was given a fifty-fifty chance of surviving surgical closure of an atrial septal defect — an operation that is now rarely, if ever, fatal.

By the 1960s, surgeons were performing coronary artery bypass operations — over 600,000 of which were performed in the United States alone last year with an operative mortality, taking all comers, of less than two in a hundred — a mortality rate less than that of gallbladder surgery. And since its introduction less that 15 years ago, cardiologists have used balloon angioplasty to relieve the pain and risk of angina for hundreds of thousands of patients with coronary artery disease who, having failed medical management, would have had no alternative to disability other than open-heart surgery.

Open-heart surgery is the success story of modern cardiovascular medicine. Surgeons now routinely correct virtually all congenital heart defects, often successfully operating on infants with hearts no larger than a kumquat. Persistent defects in the septum between the atria or the ventricles are closed either by direct suture or by a patch sewn over the defect. Ductus arteriosus — a residual connection between the pulmonary artery and the aorta — can be sewn shut. Abnormally small valves can be enlarged or in later life repaired or replaced. Complicated cyanotic heart conditions such as Tetralogy of Fallot are corrected by enlarging the inadequate pulmonic valve and sewing closed the defect in the ventricular septum, restoring the normal blood flow patterns and normal oxygenation. Very few, even rare congenital heart defects, cannot be corrected. Thousands of children each year are saved from the disability and early death that are the heritage of untreated congenital heart disease.

Life is a pyramid to which each one of us brings a stone. The success of coronary artery by-pass surgery was built on the success of by-pass operations elsewhere in the body. First developed to treat the atherosclerotic blockage of the leg blood vessels, the concept was quickly applied to blockage in the coronary arteries. The rationale for this operation is based on the fact that the blockage tends to be segmental, affecting only a short segment of the vessel. The vessel beyond the blockage is often normal.

Using a piece of vein from the leg (there is, fortunately, a double set of veins in the leg) or sometimes an artery from underneath the chest wall, a by-pass is constructed around the blockage to restore the blood flow to the area of jeopardized heart beyond. By restoring the blood flow, symptoms are relieved, and if sometime later the partial blockage becomes complete, the by-pass carries blood to the heart that would have been damaged without it.

In this way, by-pass cannot only relieve the pain of angina due to the partially-blocked vessel, but can also prevent the consequences of heart attack that would have occurred if the blockage had become complete.

Is it a perfect operation? No. Is it good for those who need it? No question about it. After years of journalistic skepticism regarding the value of coronary artery by-pass surgery, the question about by-pass is no longer whether or not it works. There is no question about that. The only question now about by-pass surgery is who needs it. It would be unethical now to redo the studies of the 1970s where patients who might benefit from by-pass surgery were randomized into either medical or surgical treatment for the purpose of study.

Coronary artery by-pass surgery is not a cure. As helpful as it has been, many problems remain. The risk of the operation remains. Even in the best of hands, surgery claims the lives of one to two percent of those it is designed to help. But this risk is more than offset by the number of lives saved and the fact that ninety-eight percent of the time, it works as it should.

Most of the deaths from cardiac surgery occur in patients in whom the risk of any type of surgery is high — older patients, those with severely damaged hearts and those with lung and kidney disease. The risk is also higher in patients with diabetes who tend to have diffuse vascular disease and in women whose vessels are smaller and technically more difficult to deal with.

Some patients who have successful cardiac surgery re-develop angina. This is sometimes due to failure of one of the grafts which may eventually occur in as many as fifteen percent of patients. But this does not mean that in those fifteen percent all of the grafts failed. If a patient with three grafted vessels loses one graft, they are still better off than they were before surgery when three vessels were bad. And closure of one graft no longer means that re-operation is required. Procedures are now available to unstop blocked grafts with catheters (angioplasty) avoiding the need for surgery.

In some patients who re-develop angina following by-pass surgery, graft failure is not the cause. All of the coronary arteries are not grafted at the time of by-pass surgery. Only the diseased ones. Disease can develop later in a vessel which was not affected at the time of surgery.

By-pass surgery is still very expensive, in large part because of the work-intensive, high-tech care which is required. And as expensive as it is, this cost must be weighed against the costs of not doing surgery when it is indicated. Almost anywhere by-pass surgery is performed, the costs are less than those incurred in treating one heart attack ($50,000) and that ignores improvements in the quality of life — which is very difficult to price — and the gains from both personal income, the resultant taxes and the worker's contribution to society.

It is very difficult to "cost account" medical care. There is much talk these days, from those who sound as if they know, about the "cost effectiveness" of treatments like cardiac surgery. It is expensive, no question. But how is the worth of a father or a wife to be determined?

The published risk of by-pass surgery varies from surgeon to surgeon and from hospital to hospital, but mortality does not tell the whole story. A surgeon can protect his "average" by operating on only low-risk patients, refusing to operate on those whose risk of dying from the surgery might be in the twenty percent range. But even these high-risk patients have an eighty percent chance of surviving, and suppose the patient — the only one whose vote really counts — is willing to accept the increased risk?

In the long run, selection of a surgeon is pretty much like everything in life. Before you sign up, ask around. Ask your personal physician. Ask your cardiologist. Consult with more than one surgeon. Seek out hospitals with institutional integrity. Picking your cardiac surgeon may be the single most important decision you make in your life. You should use at least the same diligence in picking a doctor that you would use in buying a house.

Balloon angioplasty, another method of treating coronary artery disease, was first performed by a young Swiss cardiologist in 1977. Last year in the United States alone 550,000 angioplasties were performed, about the same as the number of coronary by-pass operations. The greatest advantage of angioplasty is that partially-blocked coronary arteries can be unstopped with a fraction of the risk of open-heart surgery.

To perform this procedure, a small flexible tube or catheter about as big around as a kitchen match is inserted into an artery at the elbow or the groin through a needle stick. No surgery or general anaesthesia is required. Using x-ray fluoroscopy guidance, this tube is floated back up to the heart and threaded into the affected artery.

Attached to the end of the catheter is a tiny spherical balloon which during the insertion is deflated against the sides of the angioplasty catheter. The catheter is advanced until the balloon is at the site of the narrowing. When in place, the balloon is inflated, enlarging the narrowed artery and restoring normal blood flow. (Figure 3, see page 14)

Safer by far than open heart surgery, angioplasty nonetheless has its own risks. Occasionally the narrowing in the vessel is so severe that the balloon cannot be properly placed. Occasionally — about two cases out of a hundred — the artery is torn in the process of attempting to dilate it and urgent by-pass surgery is required. For this reason, emergency cardiac surgery backup is routinely available and can be initiated within minutes.

In more than ninety percent of cases, the angioplasty procedure is successful. A ninety percent average is pretty good in any other league. Unfortunately, modern medicine has become so miraculous, that expectations of success have been raised unrealistically high and procedures without perfect results are criticized, even when the success rate is extraordinarily high.

While angioplasty can be done on several vessels, it is usually only recommended for the treatment of patients with obstruction of one or two coronary arteries.

The main limitation of angioplasty — aside from the fact that all patients cannot be treated in this way — is that in as many of twenty-five percent of successfully treated patients, the original blockage recurs, usually within the first three months.

The popular press, with its man-bites-dog mindset has focused on this recurrence rate. They ignore, however, the fact that in the majority of patients — seventy-five percent — the procedure does not need to be repeated. And what's more, if the blockage recurs, a second dilitation is almost always successful.

Why would a procedure that has failed be repeated? The answer lies in the characteristics of the material that occludes the vessel. The material causing the original obstruction, usually hard and crusty cholesterol, is deposited in the vessel over a period of thirty to forty years. The material that develops within a few weeks after angioplasty is softer, more like soap, and this material is much more easily dilated. Hence the rationale for the repeat procedure.

In addition to balloon dilitation, obstructions within the coronary arteries can be removed by another catheter technique known as atherectomy. In this procedure, the obstructing material is pared away with a small cutting capsule or planed down with a tiny blade rotating at high speed. Both techniques are successful and have specific indications based on the nature and the location of the arterial obstruction. As with angioplasty, re-stenosis sometimes develops and the procedure must be repeated.

The cost of angioplasty — even with repeats — is less than by-pass surgery — and the risk of by-pass is 50 times higher. Patients having angioplasty or atherectomy are routinely discharged within forty-eight hours, compared to five to seven days for by-pass surgery. In almost all cases patients having angioplasty can return to work the day after they return home.

On the other hand full surgical convalescence often requires six to eight weeks depending on the patient and the occupation. It is important to point out, however, that the convalescence from cardiac surgery is to allow time for the muscles and bones of the chest wall — and not the heart itself — to heal. The site of the surgery on the heart blood vessels is healed much more quickly.

In an effort to improve the results of angioplasty and atherectomy, stents have been developed to place in the artery after the dilitation. These tiny, stainless steel culverts are placed in the artery at the site of the dilitation and splint the artery open, decreasing the chance that it will close.

Since first developed in the 1960s, corrective surgery for heart valve replacement has become commonplace. Every year thousands of heart valve replacements are performed with an average surgical mortality in the range of five percent, certainly low when the alternatives of disability or death from congestive heart failure are considered. Heart valve replacement requires open-heart surgery and can be done at the time of by-pass surgery if it is indicated.

The valves most commonly needing replacement are the aortic and the mitral valves. Some patients need both valves replaced. Risks vary considerably depending in large part on the patient's general condition. If valve replacement is delayed for too long, the pump can get burned out and replacing the valve is then of no benefit. On the other hand, replacing the valve before it is required, subjects the patient to an unnecessary risk. Expert judgment is required to time the surgery properly. Fortunately there are a number of examinations and tests to assist cardiologists and cardiac surgeons in making this critical decision.

Valve replacements are of two types — mechanical valves and tissue valves. Mechanical valves were developed first and are made of stainless steel. Tissue valves are made of animal tissue taken from pigs or human cadavers. Each has its own set of advantages and disadvantages. Prior to surgery, the surgeon will review the choices with the patient and outline the reasons for selecting either of the two types of valves.

In the vast majority of patients, valve replacement is not indicated until the patient has developed symptoms which cannot be managed with medical treatment. If it ain't broke, don't fix it!

In addition to the remarkable advances in surgical treatment of heart disease, scientists in the pharmaceutical industry have developed an impressive armamentarium of effective drugs. Hypertension and high cholesterol can now be controlled in virtually all patients. Powerful vasodilators and diuretics can relieve shortness of breath and swelling in patients with congestive heart failure, delaying, and sometimes eliminating the need for surgery.

Drugs for angina include several types of beta blockers which reduce heart rate and blood pressure, decreasing the work of the heart and allowing a heart with limited blood supply to get by with less oxygen. There is some evidence that patients treated with beta blockers after a heart attack have better long-term outcomes than those who do not receive beta blockers. Beta blockers are safe drugs which do not have any permanent adverse side effects. However, like all drugs, unpleasant side effects sometimes occur. Fatigue is perhaps the most common side effect. This is a very difficult symptom to evaluate since fatigue has so many causes. Often it is not possible to know if the beta blocker is contributing to the fatigue unless it is discontinued on a trial basis.

Coronary vasodilators, designed to maximize the blood flow to the heart, have been the mainstay treatment of coronary artery disease since nitroglycerine was found to provide temporary relief of angina. Still in use, nitroglycerine can be taken under the tongue or as an oral spray. Used in this way, the onset of action is rapid — usually within a minute — but the duration of action is short as well. Often more than one dose is required for complete relief.

Nitroglycerine is relatively harmless, and cardiologists generally encourage patients to take what nitroglycerine they need for relief. However, if the chest pain persists after two or three nitro tablets, patients are generally advised to seek medical attention, not because a larger nitro dose might be harmful, but because the persistent pain may indicate a heart attack rather than just angina. The same advice is generally given to patients who suddenly develop angina more easily, or with less exertion than usual. Angina occurring at rest or during sleep is particularly worrisome since chest pain with such minimal exertion may indicate that one of the coronary arteries is about to close off completely and cause a heart attack. This change in the pattern of angina — often referred to as unstable angina — may be a warning sign of an impending heart attack.

Nitroglycerine can be used in anticipation of activities which patients have noticed often bring on angina such as going out in the cold or walking uphill or opening the garage door. There is no specific limit to the number of nitro tablets that can be taken, but if recurrent doses are required for relief, the medical program needs to be adjusted so the pain can be prevented rather than just treated.

It is important to emphasize that angina is not just pain, but that it is a warning signal. As the blockage in the coronary artery narrows the vessel, the blood flow to part of the heart is decreased. With exercise more oxygen is needed by the heart muscle, but because of the partially blocked blood vessel, the increased oxygen demands cannot be met. This lack of oxygen makes the heart ache — the characteristic pain of angina. As the blockage increases, restricting the blood flow more and more, the ache comes on with lower and lower levels of exercise, or even emotional stress.

So angina is more than just a pain. It is an overload signal. It says that part of the heart is being asked to work without adequate oxygen. Angina says STOP. It is a sign that one or more of the heart arteries is plugging up, — a process that kills more people in the United States every year than all other causes of death put together.

While nitroglycerine is useful in relieving angina, the usual treatment is to try to prevent the angina from occurring. For this nitrates are used but in forms with more prolonged action. Nitroglycerine ointment or nitroglycerine patches can be applied to the skin once a day. The drug seeps through the skin into the blood stream in a steady dose throughout the day. Some patients develop a "resistance" to nitroglycerine; and, if so, sensitivity can be restored by removing the ointment or patch during the nighttime hours. All patients do not experience this "resistance," and many benefit from leaving the nitroglycerine on the skin throughout the day and night.

Calcium channel blockers are also very effective coronary vasodilators. These drugs interfere with the uptake of calcium by the arteries. Without calcium the muscle in the wall of the artery relaxes allowing maximum blood flow to the heart.

It is unlikely that even these powerful vasodilators can dilate thickened and diseased coronary arteries which are partially occluded by plaques of cholesterol and scar tissue. However the main coronary arteries are interconnected by a rich network of smaller collateral blood vessels, and it is these undiseased collaterals which, when dilated, can provide increased blood flow around the blockages. This collateral blood flow is sometimes adequate to relieve the symptoms of angina caused by inadequate blood supply to the portion of the heart supplied by a diseased and partially obstructed blood vessel. When it is not, angioplasty or surgery may be required to restore adequate blood flow.

It is important to emphasize that these drugs — beta blockers, nitrates, calcium channel blockers — which can be effective at lessening or relieving symptoms, do nothing to alter the basic underlying process obstructing the coronary arteries. They do not clean out the vessels like some biologic Liquid Plumber; and, as far as we know, do nothing to slow the progression of the disease. And they do nothing to reduce the risks of coronary disease. They are solely for the relief of symptoms. If relief of symptoms is the goal of treatment — and sometimes it is — medication is often adequate. If reduction of risk is the goal, the blockage in the coronary artery needs to be removed or bypassed.

Many patients with coronary disease can benefit from aspirin. Administration of aspirin is now routine for the treatment of heart attack and unstable angina. Aspirin interferes with the clumping of platelets which is thought to contribute to the formation of obstructing blood clots at the site of coronary artery narrowing. Some physicians feel that, unless specifically contraindicated, all adults should take 180 or 325 milligrams of aspirin a day. There is nothing magic about baby aspirin, which is frequently advised. It is, by comparison, quite expensive, and it is much cheaper to buy regular aspirin tablets and break them in half.

Before I leave the topic of drugs, let me clarify one source of confusion which I have found particularly frequent, that is the difference between drug *allergy* and drug *overdose*. Many patients who think they are allergic to certain drugs are not. Given enough aspirin, for instance, most patients will have a stomach ache. This is not an allergic reaction, but the predictable side effect of a large dose of aspirin. Aspirin can be irritating to the stomach. Patients' tolerances to aspirin vary, and often these side effects can be eliminated or modified by changing the dose. Aspirin allergy, on the other hand, is usually manifest, like other allergies, by rash or asthma. These allergic symptoms can occur regardless of the dose.

So when telling your doctor that you are allergic to a certain drug, make sure you are actually allergic. Otherwise, you may miss out on the potential benefits of an effective drug. If you have any questions, describe to the doctor the reaction which you thought was an allergy.

And one more thing. For those of you who read books about drugs and their adverse effects, I must point out that just because a certain side effect is possible doesn't mean you will have it. Most side effects are infrequent. You should pay careful attention to the incidence, or the chance, of having a side effect, which for most medicines is less than one in a hundred.

CHAPTER 14

GENERIC DRUGS

You Get What You Pay For

Medicines are all chemical compounds, with several aliases. Each compound has a chemical name, a generic name and a trade name. The trade name is the property of the manufacturing company, often the company that discovers it. For instance, 1,5-Benzothiazepin-4(5H) one, 3-(acetyloxy)-5-[2-(dimethylamino) ethyl]- 2-3-dihydro-2-(4-methoxyphenyl)-, monohydrochloride, (+) — cis is also known by its generic name, diltiazem, and by its trade name Cardiazem.

Cardiazem tablets are about the size of an aspirin, but only a small part of the tablet is the active ingredient. Most of the tablet is made of a filler such as lactic acid to make the tablet large enough to handle conveniently. A binder is mixed with the filler to hold it together, so it can be compressed into a tablet. This binder must be strong enough to hold the tablet together and keep it from crumbling, yet soluble enough to dissolve when swallowed. Emulsifiers are sometimes added to aid dissolving. In addition, tablets are often coated to make swallowing easier. The coating and the emulsifier can be designed to dissolve in the acid environment of the the stomach. However if the drug is irritating to the stomach, the tablet can be designed to pass through the stomach and dissolve in the alkaline environment of the small intestine.

Thus what appears on the surface to be a simple pill is actually a carefully thought out and well designed compound of several chemicals. The patent law protects the original manufacturer from any other company duplicating the drug for seven years — a period designed to allow the originator to recover the costs of research and development etc. This limited protection applies only to the active ingredient. The binder, the filler, the emulsifier and the coating are proprietary.

Tablets from two different manufacturers may contain the same amount of active ingredient and can be said to have the same bioavailability. However their effectiveness depends not only on the potential availability of the active ingredient, but whether or not the active ingredient actually gets into the blood stream. If a tablet does not dissolve properly, for instance, the active ingredient cannot get into the blood stream. Or if the tablet dissolves in the stomach rather than the small intestine it may be destroyed by the high acid content or may cause stomach irritation. The "same bioavailability" is not the same as "the same." There are simply too many variables.

A few years ago before I caught on, a patient of mine with congestive heart failure asked me one day, "Doc, are all Lasix tablets the same." Lasix is a diuretic used to relieve the fluid retention common to this condition. When I asked why, he said that he had run out of Lasix and when he refilled his prescription the druggist suggested that he could save some money by buying a generic equivalent. He took the generic tablets but quickly noticed that they were not as effective in relieving his fluid retention as the "real ones." He doubled and then tripled the dose seeking relief. Then he found some of the real Lasix which he thought he had misplaced and immediately the difference became apparent. My patients have had similar experiences with other generic drugs. One man noticed that the generic capsules he was taking for a life-threatening heart rhythm disturbance were passing undissolved in his stool.

One particularly memorable horror story involved a patient taking anticoagulants to prevent blood clots from forming on his mechanical heart valve replacement. After switching to the generic form to save money, he had a devastating stroke from a blood clot which formed on the valve and went to his brain. He was hospitalized for months at an expense of hundreds of thousands of dollars and even then was never the same. The *initial* cost of generic drugs is less, but you have to watch both sides of the ledger.

The Food and Drug Administration requires quality testing for generic drugs, but it is not the same testing required for the release of proprietary drugs. Consequently the quality varies, not only from the original manufacturer, but from one generic drug company to the other and from one batch to the other. It is ironic that in this age of "Quality Assurance," the standards for drug testing have been relaxed rather than strengthened, especially when the consequences can be so grave.

Many physicians are reluctant to prescribe generic drugs for serious medical conditions. It is one thing to prescribe generic sleeping pills or tranquilizers. If they do not work, simply increase the dose. It is quite a different matter, however, to depend on generic drugs to control life threatening seizure disorders or potentially fatal heart rhythm disturbances.

There is another issue here. Cost. Things aren't always what they seem. At one point we were considering establishing a pharmacy in our office. We realized that without the overhead of a drugstore, we could provide name brand drugs to our patients at less cost. When it occurred to us that we might be criticized for not providing generic drugs, I checked more carefully into the drug pricing. What I found was surprising.

A hundred Lasix tablets, for instance, might sell for $40. A hundred generic Lasix might sell for $20. Assuming the drugs are actually therapeutically equal, that seems like a pretty good deal. But what interested me the most was the druggist's mark-up. The one hundred Lasix cost the druggist $36, so his profit was $4. However the druggist's cost for the one hundred generic Lasix was $5, so the profit was $15. That is not to say that druggists recommend generic drugs to pad their own pockets, but there is certainly a conflict of interest.

More and more managed care organizations require that physicians prescribe generic drugs when available. If this happens to you, discuss with your physician the potential consequences and do not hesitate to request a brand-name drug if you have any doubts — especially if the medical condition is a potentially dangerous one. If the physician cannot or will not prescribe a brand-name drug, I would consider asking the advice of another physician. Those who encourage second opinions regarding certain surgical treatments should not be resistant to second opinions for medical treatments as well.

All the same, you might say, spare the guys a little profit if the patient can save some money too. But that reasoning assumes the products are the same.

When you get right down to it, nothing much has changed. There is no free lunch. You get pretty much what you pay for. So for the buyer of generic drugs I have only one bit of advice . . . LET THE BUYER BEWARE.

Chapter 15

PREVENTION: WHAT CAN I DO TO HELP?
Good Fat, Bad Fat Or Can Diet Do It?

The prevention of heart disease is the great hope of modern medicine. The need for prevention is paramount. Heart disease, once developed, can be disabling; and too often there is no warning that it is about to strike. For many the first symptom of heart disease is the last. As many as half of all first cardiac events end in death and those who survive are five times more likely than normal to die within five years.

Efforts to prevent heart disease have been directed largely at the prevention of coronary artery disease or heart attack. Heart attack is caused by blockage of one or more than one of the coronary arteries, but the underlying cause of this artery disease is not known.

What is known is that this artery disease is segmental — that is, only certain areas of the artery develop disease. The blockage does not extend throughout the length of the vessel but is limited to short segments of the vessels, as if they had been crimped with pliers. This has led to the development of coronary artery by-pass surgery to by-pass this blockage and to angioplasty to dilate this blockage. (Figure 3, see page 14)

It is also known that certain factors seem to contribute to the development of coronary artery disease prematurely or more rapidly. These so-called risk factors include diabetes, high cholesterol, cigarette smoking, high blood pressure and obesity.

There appears to be some genetic predisposition as well, since some people who have coronary artery disease in their family, seem to do everything right but still have heart attacks.

One popular theory holds that something damages the inner lining of the heart artery; and that, in an attempt to repair the damage done to this blood vessel, the body piles up scar tissue where blood fats (which usually pass through the arterial lining) accumulate. This partial blockage creates eddy currents which somehow lead to further efforts at repair and plaque formation. As the plaque builds up, the blood flow is critically limited to a certain part of the heart and angina develops. If the remaining channel becomes too narrow, and the blood flow slows enough, a blood clot may develop, blocking the final pinpoint opening. This process forms the basis for the treatment with thrombolytic agents such as t-Pa, agents which dissolve the clot.

Others feel that the plaque may actually tear partially loose from the arterial wall forming a flap that occludes the blood flow and causes a heart attack.

The cause of this scourge is not yet known, but several so-called risk factors have been identified which, when present, seem to increase the likelihood of developing heart disease. Current efforts to prevent heart disease are based on recognition and control of the risk factors.

The most important of these risk factors are related to life-style, such as high fat diet, smoking, high blood pressure and diabetes. The role of these factors has been established by years of medical research, including clinical and pathological investigation, animal experimentation and epidemiological research. Attention to and modification of these risk factors — especially control of high blood pressure and cholesterol — may have contributed to the twenty-two percent decrease in coronary artery disease (CAD) mortality over the past ten years.

The chance of developing coronary disease increases with age and is higher in men than women, but this is not subject to control. Of those risk factors that can be controlled, blood cholesterol may be the most important.

Epidemiologic studies have been remarkably consistent in indicating a relationship between high serum cholesterol and the incidence of CAD. In addition, the risk is directly related to the level of cholesterol in the blood. For those with cholesterol levels of over 260, the risk of developing CAD is four times that of those with cholesterol levels of 170. Thus the higher the cholesterol, the greater the risk. This risk is independent of other risk factors such as smoking, hypertension and diabetes.

The safe level of cholesterol is not known but studies have indicated that the risk of CAD increased markedly with serum cholesterol levels over 180.

Cholesterol is made up of two main components which can be separated chemically — and the risk of high cholesterol is related to the proportion of these two components.

The so-called "good" cholesterol is high density lipoprotein (HDL) which usually comprises about twenty-five percent of the cholesterol in the blood. "Bad" cholesterol, or low density lipoprotein (LDL) makes up the other seventy-five percent. Studies have shown that for any given level of cholesterol, the higher the proportion of LDL, the greater the risk of developing CAD.

A serum cholesterol test measures total cholesterol and is of some value. More valuable, however, is an analysis which measures the total cholesterol as well as the percent of each of the two fractions. Both tests are readily available. It is important that these tests be done in the fasting state — with nothing to eat for at least twelve hours. Testing the blood shortly after eating can show falsely elevated cholesterol levels.

In most patients reducing the amount of cholesterol in the diet can lower the blood cholesterol level. Weight reduction can also be helpful and is usually the first order of business for overweight patients. Most dietary cholesterol comes from animal fat — such as beef, pork and dairy products such as eggs, milk, butter and cheese.

Blood cholesterol can also be reduced by limiting the amount of saturated fat in the diet. These saturated fats are thought to be particularly liable to raise the blood cholesterol levels.

The term "saturated" refers to the chemical structure of the fat and indicates that binding sites for hydrogen on the fat molecule are saturated. This saturation with hydrogen gives the fat a higher melting point. Unsaturated fats, which are less likely to raise the blood cholesterol, have a lower melting point and most are liquid at room temperature giving rise to the adage that if you can pour it, you can eat it. Exceptions are the tropical oils, such as coconut oil which, though liquid, are highly saturated.

Current dietary recommendations include restricting daily cholesterol intake to no more than 300 milligrams — the amount contained in a breakfast of scrambled eggs, sausage and hash brown potatoes. *Total* fat for the average size middle-aged person should be no more than thirty percent of total calories (about 80 grams per day) — 3.5 ounces of Macadamia nuts or two helpings of cheese tortellini Alfredo. Compliance with these restrictions requires some study of the fat content of foods. The new federal labeling system should help with this task.

A number of excellent diet books are available. Common sense and moderation should prevail. It makes no sense to severely restrict dietary fat in an effort to lower cholesterol if the diet is one that cannot be sustained for life. Do the best that you can, and then check your cholesterol to see how you're doing. The serum cholesterol changes slowly so frequent checks are unnecessary.

Diet is only one source of the cholesterol in the blood. Cholesterol is manufactured by the liver. It is a necessary precursor for a variety of chemicals needed by the body. As with other biologic processes, some people make more cholesterol that others. Those whose bodies make large amounts of cholesterol cannot reduce their blood cholesterol levels to the recommended level even if they ate no cholesterol or fat at all. These people will need drugs to help them. Diet is the first thing to try. If it is not effective, medicine can help.

Fortunately, a number of drugs are now available which can markedly reduce blood cholesterol levels, often to normal. This is something we could not say ten or even five years ago. It is important to emphasize that these drugs are not a cure, like penicillin is for pneumonia. They lower cholesterol only as long as they are in the system. Once the drug is discontinued, the cholesterol will return to the pre-treatment level. As we now understand it, if cholesterol-lowering drugs of some type are ever required, they will be required for life.

In addition to cholesterol, triglyceride is another type of fat in the blood that can contribute to the development of coronary artery disease. Triglyceride levels can be measured in the blood and these determinations are routinely included in the fractional analysis of blood lipids or fats.

In contrast to blood cholesterol which can be elevated by increased fat intake, blood triglycerides are elevated by carbohydrate — especially sugar and alcohol — intake. Serum triglyceride levels are particularly sensitive to changes in body weight and sometimes impressive reductions in serum triglycerides can be achieved by weight loss alone, thereby avoiding the need for medicine. For those whose triglyceride remains elevated even after reducing to normal body weight, a number of effective drugs are available.

Dietary fat is not only the main source of fat in the blood, it is the main source of calories. Fat contains seven calories per gram, more than twice the number of calories in a gram of either sugar or protein. So a low fat diet is not only a low-cholesterol diet, it is also a weight reduction diet. In this way a low-fat diet can lower the triglyceride as well.

Unfortunately fat is also the source of much of the taste in food. After describing the low fat diet to a pragmatic old Maine Downeaster I asked him if he understood my instructions. "Yep," came the reply. "If it tastes good, spit it out."

As sad as it is, a low-fat diet takes some adjustment, especially after a lifetime of rich American food But it comes under the heading of preventive maintenance, much like changing the oil in your car. Having a high blood cholesterol and trigylceride is like driving around with dirty oil in the car. It is all too common to find people, religiously changing the oil in their cars, who have never had their cholesterol checked.

A second major risk factor for coronary artery disease is high blood pressure, the most common of all cardiovascular disorders, affecting fifty million people in the United States. The increased risk of high blood pressure is related to both the amount the pressure is elevated and the length of time it has been present. The risk is increased by elevations of either the systolic or the diastolic blood pressure.

In patients with diastolic blood pressures (the bottom number of the recording) in the range of 90-100 mm Hg — so-called "mild" hypertension — the risk of developing coronary artery disease is doubled, and tripled for those with diastolic pressures of 110-115. In one study of men age thirty-five to fifty-seven, nearly thirty percent had elevated diastolic blood pressure.

The risks of elevated systolic blood pressure (the upper number of the recording) are similar. There is a progressive risk of developing coronary artery disease with systolic blood pressure of over 130 mm Hg, even if the diastolic blood pressure is normal. At systolic blood pressures of 140-145, the risk of coronary artery disease doubles and for those with systolic blood pressures in the 175-180 range, the risk is increased eight fold.

In these times there is no excuse for having high blood pressure. Detection is simple and cheap, and with a host of effective drugs available, control is essentially always possible. Like high blood cholesterol, however, treating high blood pressure is a lifetime treatment. Medicine can control it, but only as long as it is being taken. You never "get over" high blood pressure. It can be controlled, but never cured.

Many studies have demonstrated that cigarette smoking is directly related to an increased risk of developing coronary artery disease, heart attack and sudden death. The overall risk of developing coronary disease is twice as high for smokers as it is for patients who do not smoke. It is no accident that life insurance underwriters charge smokers higher premiums. Those smokers trying to quit may find it encouraging that within two years of quitting, the risk of coronary artery disease returns to normal.

The exact mechanism by which smoking produces the increased risk is not yet known. One theory has it that smoking contributes to increased stickiness of blood platlets. These little particles circulate in the blood and plug up the hundreds of little unseen breaks in blood vessels which we sustain each day, much as Never-Leak plugs holes in faulty car radiators. Smoking makes these platelets more adhesive, causing them to pile up at the site of these sealed leaks in masses that eventually block off the blood vessel entirely. Whether or not this is entirely true, it is a graphic way to think about it. Smoking makes the blood sludgy.

For both men and women with diabetes, the risk of coronary artery disease is increased 4.8 and 5.8 times respectively. Some of this excess risk may be due to the elevated levels of cholesterol and triglyceride, levels which can usually be reduced with diet, good control of the diabetes and drugs if necessary.

While each of these risk factors can independently influence the odds of developing coronary artery disease, combinations of risk factors are even more dangerous. Thus for a cigarette smoking hypertensive man with a serum cholesterol of 245, the risk of developing coronary artery disease is increased thirteen times! If this man quit smoking, his risk drops to six times normal. If he then decreased his cholesterol to 200, his risk drops to twice normal. And if he then controls his blood pressure, his risk drops to normal.

Studies in several countries have shown an association between sedentary life style and an increased risk of developing coronary artery disease. The mechanism for this is not known, and there is much discussion about how much exercise — and what kind — is required to neutralize the risk. Until this is settled, it would be prudent to build some sort of regular exercise into our lives.

Any exercise helps muscle tone. It also burns calories and can help with weight reduction. For cardiovascular benefit, exercises which increase heart rate are probably best, so-called aerobic exercise. In simple terms that means that the exercise should produce some shortness of breath.

It is recommended that at least once a day we increase the heart rate moderately and then maintain that increase for twenty minutes. Exercises such as walking outside or on a treadmill, swimming or riding a stationary bicycle are good ones. The outdoor bicycle riding I have seen appears to be mostly coasting. Walking is the cheapest and the most available exercise and can be modified to suit almost everyone. Studies have demonstrated that walking at three miles per hour one to three hours a week reduces the risk of heart disease by as much as thirty percent!

The most fortunate of us live close enough to work to walk. This satisfies our American passion to be accomplishing more than one thing at a time. For those who live too far to walk, how about a Park-and-Walk plan? Drive to within a mile of work, park and walk the rest of the way.

Running or jogging is good exercise, but not suitable for those of us with older joints. If you want to try jogging, get the best shoes you can afford and don't run on the pavement. Find some grass or a track.

I have met only a few who could maintain an interest in swimming. The trips to the pool and the clothes changes take a lot of time, and often there is a fee. Almost any type of exercise equipment is good if it produces some shortness of breath, provided you can maintain the pace for the required twenty minutes. Equipment that exercises the upper body as well as the lower body is preferable.

The trouble, of course, is that exercise takes time. It is difficult for busy people, who already think time is short, to set aside time for exercising. Diligence is required. It has to be built into the day. Each person has his own solution. I have one patient who sleeps in his sweat suit. When the alarm goes off he goes out to walk, and on the way through the kitchen hits the switch on the automatic coffee pot which takes nine minutes to brew. He walks briskly for ten minutes — not perfect, but better than nothing — and on passing back through the kitchen he picks up a cup of coffee and takes it upstairs to begin his day. Typical American solution. No wasted time or motion.

Formal exercise programs are best for some who need the motivation — and can make the time. Sometimes just paying dues at the local YMCA or buying a treadmill or indoor bike is enough of an incentive. "Got to get my money's worth." But other options are available. How about parking as far, rather than as close to work as possible? How about seeking out stairs to walk — up and down — rather than use the elevator? Every little bit helps.

I am amused to see people who avoid stairs at work and at home, yet go to a gym and pay money to walk on the Stairmaster. Human nature, I suppose.

One word of caution. Those planning to begin an exercise program, especially if they are middle-aged or over, should seriously consider having an exercise test. It may uncover unsuspected heart disease that would make exercising dangerous. Some will argue that an exercise test is unnecessary, even expensive, but all things are relative. Others will argue that it is prudent. You would have your car checked out before a long road trip, wouldn't you?

There is a lot of hear-say to suggest that vitamin E is somehow good for the cardiovascular system and that it may even help prevent coronary artery disease. A recent study has claimed that vitamin E is the beneficial element in the Mediterranean diet that has been sought for so long. Doctors have varying degrees of conviction about the benefits of vitamin E, but since the risk of moderate doses (400U per day) is certainly low and the benefits may be real, it seems worth the risk.

Does alcohol reduce the risk or developing coronary artery disease? Wine drinkers rejoiced at the news that moderate use of red wine appears to prolong the lives of Frenchmen, even in the face of what some would consider a rich diet. However, recent data from America suggested that while four drinks a week provided some protection against developing heart disease, a drink a day did not. Vive la difference!

And what about coffee? Who knows?

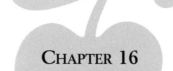

CHAPTER 16

STRESS:

Is It Really Worth Dying For?

Is it having to increase your sales every year? Is it a crying baby on an airplane? Is it unpaid bills? Traffic jams or taxes? Thankless children? Chronic pain? Time pressure? Telephones?

What drives one person to distraction might roll off another like water off a duck's back. I watched my grandfather, who lived to be ninety-four, struggle against the cruel vagaries of weather and economics trying to save his East Texas farm. But sometimes it's not the big things, but the little things that seem the sharpest. I remember telling him once that I was afraid of tigers. I can still see his face and hear his soothing voice as he patted me on the hand and said, "It's not the tigers that'll get 'cha Son, it's the gnats."

Stress has many important effects on the body. It can release adrenalin, raising the state of alertness, the heart rate and the blood pressure, readying us for flight of fight. But just how this reaction could lead to cardiovascular disease is still a mystery.

Although many courts have been called to rule on the issue, the role of stress as a cause of heart disease has never been established. We lack a way of measuring stress. There are no units of measure. And there is no way to measure the effect of stress on a person, let alone his heart. And while it seems logical in some ways that stress can break your heart, until we have some scientific data, we simply have to say that the role of stress as a cause of heart disease is purely conjectural.

For the reader who would like to know more about what is known about stress, I would recommend the the fine book by cardiologist Robert Eliot, *Is It Worth Dying For* (Bantam Books).

CHAPTER 17

SECOND OPINIONS

In a word, GET ONE. If your doctor is balky about helping you get a second opinion, get a new doctor.

He should have been sensitive enough to your needs to sense you were uneasy and wanted to ask someone else's advice before you had to ask. He should know that even before you asked him about a second opinion, that you had agonized about whether or not to ask. Agonized about whether or not to risk hurting his feelings or pride by asking for another opinion. Agonized about the uncertainty in not asking. He should have suggested it before you had to.

Often the best source of a second opinion is your personal doctor. Ask him what he thinks of the specialist's recommendations. Just because you ask for a second opinion does not mean you have lost confidence in the doctor or do not trust him. Opinions differ, especially in a scientific art such as medicine.

If you are uneasy about any aspect of the planned course of management you should ask someone else's advice. You would do it with a house mortgage. Or a college for your children. Why not your health? And there probably won't be a difference of opinion. Perhaps the second doctor can just explain it better.

It is just as important to ask for a second opinion about a plan that is recommended as it is to ask about a plan which is discouraged. And remember it is not your doctor's job to make the decision for you. It is your doctor's job to explain the plan to you and make sure you understand it well enough for you to make the decision.

One of the many things I learned from my father about the practice of medicine was to "always beat the patient to the consult." It insures the best treatment and preserves his confidence in you.

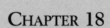

CHAPTER 18

BY-PASS SURGERY

So You Have Had By-pass Surgery. Now What?

Coronary artery by-pass surgery works. There can be no question about that. Just ask someone whose angina has been relieved. Does it work every time? No, but what does?

Whether or not, and how well cardiac surgery succeeds depends more than anything else on what the surgeon is given to work with. A heart that is ruined beyond repair cannot be fixed. It is not any easier to make a silk purse out of a sow's ear in medicine than it is in the garment trade.

If a heart has been destroyed by heart attacks, or if the coronary arteries are too severely diseased, it is not likely that an operation will be much of a success.

Whether any enterprise is judged successful depends on the goals set. What are physicians trying to accomplish here, anyway? If heart surgery is undertaken in an attempt to save or prolong life, the patient who stands to have his life saved may accept a relatively high risk of failure. If on the other hand, as with a hip replacement, heart surgery is undertaken to relieve intractable pain which cannot be otherwise controlled, the patient may not be willing to accept much risk. Thus the risk that the patient is willing to accept depends on what he thinks he has to gain. What is the risk and what is the benefit? The success of a heart operation cannot be judged by the neat figures on tables of averages, but on an individual basis. The physician's contract is still with the individual patient.

By any analysis coronary by-pass surgery is amazingly successful. The disabling chest pain of angina is uniformly relieved, many patients are saved from almost certain heart attack and all at a risk of dying (taking all comers) of less that three percent — about half the risk of having your gall bladder out.

In general, when successful, physicians consider coronary artery surgery a complete fix. We have not deluded ourselves into believing that it is a cure for coronary artery disease; but we have fixed what we have found and we urge patients who have had successful surgery to return to a normal life style without any restrictions or limitations.

Do some patients who have had heart surgery develop more coronary disease later? Yes. Coronary artery by-pass surgery does not prevent coronary artery disease, but it does give many a second chance they would not otherwise have had. And they should capitalize on that chance and plan for a normal life, taking care to do what they can to prevent or slow down the development of further disease. Why waste time dreading the possibilities? The glass is half full. Get on with it.

CHAPTER 19

HEART DISEASE IN WOMEN

~

That women get heart disease should come as no surprise. Women are subject to every form of heart disease described in this book. The surprise is that for so long women did not seem to get heart disease. Then something changed. Women began having heart attacks. For a long time this was not recognized. During my medical training in the 60s it was conventional wisdom that if a woman came to the emergency room complaining of chest pain, whatever it was, it was not a heart attack.

Since we don't know why men have heart attacks, we don't know why women have heart attacks. Many theories have been advanced to explain the marked increase in heart attack among women which began near the end of WW II. Their increase in smoking and the stress modern women are exposed to, are a couple of possibilities. But the fact remains that we do not know any more about why women have heart attacks than why men do.

What we do know is that heart disease is now the leading killer of women. Let me say that again. Heart disease is the most common cause of death in women — three times more common than breast cancer.

In the past few years, heart disease in women has become so common that there is no reluctance among experienced and well-trained physicians to consider the diagnosis of heart disease in women. It is simply too well known. I share the impression of those who suggest that women may delay seeking medical attention longer than men. This delay sometimes means that the condition has advanced farther than in men by the time they are seen. To some extent that is a failure to communicate to women — preoccupied by the fear of breast cancer — that heart disease is an even greater risk.

In addition to avoiding the usual risk factors, there is one special thing that women can do to reduce their risk of coronary artery disease. Recent studies have demonstrated a lower incidence of coronary artery disease among post-menopausal women taking low dosages of estrogen. There are some risks associated with estrogen therapy, but the preponderance of evidence now suggests that estrogen replacement is a good idea. Each patient is different, and women who are considering taking advantage of the protection estrogen replacement offers should seek their physician's advice.

Some studies have suggested that the results of by-pass surgery are not as good in women as in men. Part of this is due to the fact that the disease is often more advanced — and harder to fix — when women seek attention. Part of the reason, however, is a mechanical one. Women have smaller coronary arteries than men. Smaller arteries are harder to work with than large ones and they are harder to sew properly, so the results of surgery are sometimes not as good.

Perhaps in time surgical techniques can be improved to the point that they are not so size sensitive. In the meantime it's all the more necessary for women to become aware that they are not immune from the epidemic of heart disease. They should learn the warning signs of heart trouble and seek medical attention at the earliest sign of trouble. Better yet they should work with their physicians to participate in early detection of heart disease with the same diligence and enthusiasm that they seek early signs of breast cancer. Both are deadly.

CHAPTER 20

CARDIOLOGISTS

Just What Are Cardiologists And What Is It That They Do?

C ardiologists are medical specialists who limit their practice to the diagnosis and management of patients who have, or are suspected of having, heart disease.

In their role as consultants, they often serve to assist general physicians, providing them and their patients with advice about the diagnosis and treatment of heart disease.

Many cardiologists provide a number of specialized procedures for which they have been specifically trained, but much of the time that cardiologists spend with patients is devoted to diagnosing the patient's condition by examining their hearts and extracting the details of their medical history. Cardiologists do not perform cardiac surgery, but do play an important role in determining who might benefit from surgery, if needed, and in providing medical care and reassurance for those who do not.

The medical specialty of cardiology was not created by cardiologists. Specialty medicine was created by the United States government during World War II in an effort to provide the best possible medical care for those in the armed services. Since that time the growth of medical specialization has been driven by the rapid expansion of medical knowledge and the need for physicians with the special skills to apply it. The growth of medical specialties is, in many ways, merely another reflection of the general societal trend toward specialization as a means of coping with a burgeoning knowledge base.

The training of a cardiologist is intensive and long. Following four years of medical school, physicians who would be cardiologists enter a two year period of postgraduate training in general internal medicine studying the diseases of adults. Upon completion of this training and after certification by the American Board of Internal Medicine, those candidates who are selected (qualify) for cardiology training spend a minimum of three years — sometimes five — studying diseases of the heart. During this time they are also trained to perform and interpret a number of special examinations including electrocardiograms, echocardiograms, pacemaker evaluations, stress tests, nuclear cardiology imaging and cardiac catheterization. Some elect to spend an additional year or two learning specialized techniques for implantation of permanent pacemakers and theraputic techniques such as radiofrequency ablation of cardiac rhythm disturbances, coronary balloon angioplasty and atherectomy.

After completing this training those who pass a rigorous two-day examination are certified by the American Board of Internal Medicine Subspecialty Board of Cardiovascular Diseases. Only those cardiologists who complete the required training and pass the qualifying examination are entitled to refer to themselves as Board Certified Cardiologists. In the United States, only about ten percent of those who designate themselves as cardiologists are actually Board Certified.

Those cardiologists who are Board Certified and have practiced two years may, upon recommendation of their peers, apply for Fellowship in the American College of Cardiology. Successful candidates are awarded the designation Fellow of the American College of Cardiology, and in recognition of their achievement are allowed to use the initials F.A.C.C. after their name. It is advisable to look for this designation when selecting a cardiologist.

Of the approximately 650,000 physicians in the United States, three percent, or 20,000, are Fellows of the American College of Cardiology, and their names are listed in the Directory of Medical Specialists.

Although cardiologists do perform a number of valuable diagnostic and theraputic procedures, much of the care provided by cardiologists is what is now fashionably called "cognitive". This care begins with a careful interview and a physical examination with special emphasis on the cardiovascular system. The examination begins as patients sit across the desk talking. Patients are carefully interrogated for clues in their medical history which may indicate the presence of heart disease. Like other physicians, cardiologists are trained observers and take note during the interview of any external evidence of heart disease such as skin color, breathing patterns and external deformities which may indicate structural heart malformations or malfunction. The interview is followed by an examination of the cardiovascular system which includes determination of the blood pressure, inspection of the veins and arteries in the neck, examination of the pulses in the arms and legs, examination of the lungs and a thorough listen to the heart for abnormalities of heart rhythm, heart murmurs or extra heart sounds. Often an accurate cardiac diagnosis can be made on the basis of the medical history and the examination alone. It is the cardiologist's special skill at performing and interpreting the cardiovascular examination that perhaps most of all distinguishes them from other physicians, and it is for this that their opinion is most often sought when dealing with heart disease.

Cardiologists are also skilled at knowing which — if any — confirmatory tests are needed, and which ones are likely to be the most helpful. In this way, seeking the advice of a cardiologist can not only be the most accurate approach to caring for a patient suspected of having heart disease but can also be the most economical since the testing is the most appropriate and unnecessary duplication or repetition is avoided.

Not every patient with heart disease needs a cardiologist. In many cases the care provided by a general physician is perfectly satisfactory. However one of the most valuable things a general physician learns during training is how to make the best use of specialists and at times cardiologists can be especially helpful. The most important thing is to have the right doctor at the right time.

EPILOGUE

∿

The main message about the treatment of heart disease is that there is always hope. No matter in what condition patients with heart disease find themselves, there is always hope that treatment for their condition is, or will become available.

Just look back at the remarkable progress made by medical science in the past twenty-five years. Surgical correction of congenital heart defects. Coronary artery by-pass surgery. Artificial heart valve replacements. Implantable pacemakers and defibrillators. Coronary angioplasty and atherectomy and stent placement. Powerful and effective drugs for the treatment of hypertension, congestive heart failure, hypercholesterolemia and heart rhythm disturbances.

And the progress continues. A recent report indicates that coronary artery disease may be caused by an infection. If this is true, not only will medical scientists develop a cure for heart disease, but they will also develop a vaccine; and, in time, heart attack will be as rare as whooping cough is today.

GLOSSARY

~

Acute: Of recent or sudden onset.

Angina pectoris (or angina): Pain originating in the heart, caused by one or more narrowed blood vessels which limit the blood flow to part of the heart making it "ache".

Angiogram: A test which uses contrast material (or "dye") injected into the circulation to make the blood vessels or heart chambers visible by x-ray.

Angioplasty: Opening a narrowed or blocked blood vessel by inflating within the narrowing a small balloon attached to the end of a catheter.

Anticoagulation: Using drugs — anticoagulants — to reduce the ability of the blood to form clots.

Aorta: The main blood vessel (artery) leading from the heart.

Aortic valve: The valve between the heart and the aorta.

Arrhythmia: Abnormal heart rhythm.

Arteries: Blood vessels which carry blood from the heart.

Arteriosclerosis (or atherosclerosis): The process that thickens the walls of arteries leading to their obstruction.

Atherectomy: Opening a narrowed or blocked artery with a small, high-speed, rotary cutting blade attached to the end of a catheter.

Atrial septal defect: A congenital heart defect in which the hole in the atrial septum normally present before birth does not close after birth.

Atrium: One of two — left and right — "booster pumps" for the ventricles.

Bradycardia: Slow heart beat.

Beta-blockers: A class of drugs which blocks the effects of adrenaline. Used to treat many conditions including angina and high blood pressure.

Calcium channel blockers: Vasodilator drugs used to treat angina and high blood pressure.

Cardiomyopathy: A weakening of the heart muscle.

Cardiovascular disease: Conditions affecting the heart and blood vessels.

Cardioversion: Converting an abnormal heart rhythm to normal, using drugs (chemical cardioversion) or electric shock, applied to the chest (external cardioversion) or to the inside of the heart with a catheter (internal cardioversion).

Catheter: A small, hollow, flexible tubing inserted into the vascular system by way of a blood vessel for the purpose of measuring pressure, injecting "dye", or opening an obstruction. (see angioplasty, atherectomy).

Catheterization: The process of inserting a catheter into the vascular system by way of a blood vessel for the the purpose of measuring pressure, performing angiography, angioplasty or atherectomy.

Chronic: Of long duration.

Cholesterol: A chemical manufactured by the liver and found in animal tissue.

Congenital heart disease: A heart defect which occurs during the development of the infant before birth.

Congestive heart failure: A term used to indicate that the heart is not pumping blood as efficiently as it should. In advanced cases excess fluid accumulate in the lungs (congestion).

Coronary arteries: Arteries (two main ones — left and right — with branches) which arise from the aorta and deliver blood to the heart muscle.

Coronary angiogram (or coronary arteriogram): The motion picture record of the coronary arteries.

Coronary angiography (or coronary arteriography): X-ray photography of the coronary arteries which have been transiently filled with "dye," using a catheter, to make them visible.

Cyanosis (cyanotic): Term used to describe the bluish appearance of skin supplied by blood without adequate oxygen. Some forms of congenital heart disease produce cyanosis.

Defibrillator (see Cardioversion): An electric device which delivers a shock to the heart to stop an abnormal heart rhythm. "External" defibrillators apply the shock to the outside of the chest. "Internal" defibrillators apply the shock to the inside of the heart. For abnormal heart rhythms which occur frequently "internal" defibrillators are implanted under the skin.

Diastole: Relaxation (with filling) of the heart chambers.

Digitalis: A drug used to strengthen the heart contraction and regulate the heart rhythm.

Diuretics (or "water pills"): A class of drugs used to rid the body of excess salt (sodium) and water.

Drug trial: Evaluating the effects of a drug or drugs in treating a condition.

Echocardiography: A non-invasive technique that uses ultra-sound (radar) to study the heart.

Edema: A term which refers to swelling, usually of the feet and legs, due to excess fluid in the body.

Electrocardiogram (or EKG or ECG): A record of the electrical activity of the heart. Used to detect abnormal heart rhythm, damage to the heart or abnormal heart development.

Electrophysiologic study: Study of abnormal heart rhythms using recordings made from inside the heart with a catheter. An electrocardiogram recorded from inside the heart.

Endocardium: The ultra-thin, cellophane-like membrane that lines the inside of the heart, including the surface of the valves.

Endocarditis: Infection or inflamation of the endocardium, usually that lining the valves.

Femoral artery: The artery to the leg which is used as an entry point for inserting a catheter into the circulation.

Fibrillation: (atrial or ventricular) Chaotic or disorganized contraction of a heart chamber that reduces its ability to pump blood. Ventricular fibrillation — fibrillation of the main pumping chamber — is very dangerous. Atrial fibrillation — fibrillation of the "booster pump" — is not.

Generic drugs: Drugs of a certain general class; i.e., vasodilator drugs, but those without the brand name or trademark of a specific company. Aspirin is a generic drug. Bayer Aspirin is not.

Graft: Term used to describe the surgical attachment of one blood vessel to another to by-pass a blood vessel narrowed or blocked by plaque, as in coronary artery by-pass graft.

Heart Attack: A term often used to refer to the heart damage which occurs when an artery to part of the heart becomes blocked.

Heart Failure (see Congestive Heart Failure): A term used to indicate that the heart is not pumping blood as efficiently as it should.

Holter recording: A battery-operated device worn externally which records the electrocardiogram for several hours.

Hypertension: Abnormally high blood pressure.

Innocent heart murmur: A noise produced within the heart or blood vessels which is not thought to be due to an abnormality

Internal mammary artery: The artery — left and right — running along and underneath each side of the breast bone (sternum) sometimes used as a graft to by-pass a blocked or narrowed coronary artery.

Invasive procedure: Refers to a procedure which requires small incisions in the skin, usually to insert a catheter into a blood vessel.

Lipids (or lipoproteins): Fats including cholesterol, high density (HDL) and low density (LDL) lipoproteins and triglycerides which circulate in the blood.

mm Hg: Traditional method of expressing blood pressure as the number of millimeters (mm) which a column of mercury (Hg) is raised. Normal blood pressure is, for example 140 (mm Hg) over 80 (mmHg).

Mitral valve: Heart valve between the left atrium and the left ventricle.

Mitral valve prolapse: A condition in which one of the mitral valve leaflets bulges back (prolapses) into the atrium during the heart beat.

Murmur: Noise produced by blood flow — sometimes abnormal — within the heart or blood vessels. Detected by use of a stethoscope.

Myocardial infarction (see Heart Attack): Death (infarction) of part of the heart muscle (myocardium) resulting from a blocked artery.

Myocarditis: Infection or inflamation of the myocardium.

Myocardium: Heart muscle.

Nitroglycerine: A vasodilator drug absorbed from the mouth or through the skin used in its short-acting form to relieve angina, and in its long acting form to prevent it.

Non-invasive: Refers to a procedure which does not require a skin incision — such as an electrocardiogram or an echocardiogram.

Pacemaker: May refer to the heart's natural pacemaker, where the heart rhythm originates, or to an artificial pacemaker used to electrically stimulate a normal heart rhythm when the heart's natural pacemaker is not functioning properly.

Palpitation: The sensation felt by the patient of an abnormal heart rhythm.

Perfusion scan (see Thallium scan): A procedure which uses a small dose of radioactive chemical to study the blood flow to the heart muscle.

Pericarditis: Infection or inflamation of the pericardium.

Pericardium: Literally "around the heart." A sack of leather-like tissue enveloping the heart like a sock.

Plaque: Term for the material accumulating in the arterial wall which narrows or blocks it.

Pulmonary artery: The artery leading from the right ventricle to the lungs.

Pulmonary valve (or pulmonic valve): The heart valve between the right ventricle and the lungs.

Radiofrequency: A source of energy used to destroy the source of an abnormal heart rhythm.

Rheumatic fever: An infection which could sometimes, but often did not, damage one or more of the heart valves.

Saturated fats: Fats whose chemical composition does not allow them to be liquid at room temperature. (i.e. lard)

Septum: Tissue division, or partition, separating two chambers of the heart; i.e., atrial septum or ventricular septum.

xStenosis: Term to indicate narrowing of a blood vessel by plaque.

Stent: A small, short tube of flexible mesh which can be inserted inside a vessel — like a tiny culvert — to keep the vessel open following angioplasty or atherectomy.

Stress test: A test in which the heart is stressed — usually using exercise on a treadmill or stationary bicycle — to uncover the effects of blocked or narrowed heart blood vessels not apparent at rest.

Supraventricular: Literally "above the ventricle," referring to a rhythm disturbance originating in the atrium.

Systole: Contraction (with emptying) of the heart chambers.

Tachycardia: Rapid heart beat.

Tetralogy of Fallot: The most common cyanotic congenital heart condition, named for Dr. Fallot who described it. A persistence of the fetal heart circulation after birth.

Thallium scan: A stress test which uses a small dose of radioactive chemical (thallium) to demonstrate areas of heart muscle where the blood supply is not adequate due to a narrowed or blocked coronary artery.

Thrombolysis: The use of drugs to dissolve blood clots.

Thrombolytic drugs: Drugs used to dissolve blood clots.

Tricuspid valve: Three-leafed heart valve between the right atrium and the right ventricle.

Triglyceride: One of the lipids (fats) circulating in the blood.

Unsaturated fats: Fats whose chemical composition allows them to be liquid at room temperature; ie, oils.

Vasodilators: A class of drugs used to relax blood vessels and lower blood pressure.

Veins: Blood vessels which carry blood back to the heart.

Ventricle: One of two — left and right — muscular pumping chambers of the heart.

Ventricular septal defect: A congenital heart defect in which the hole normally present in the ventricular septum before birth does not close after birth.

Ventriculogram: A motion picture of the beating heart obtained by injecting "dye" or x-ray contrast into the ventricle through a catheter.

This is *the* book for the layman who wants to understand heart disease and its treatment.

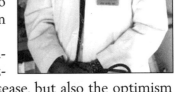

Dr. Wise presents a balanced and reasonable overview of the more common medical conditions affecting the heart in the clear and simple language that, during his thirty years of cardiology practice, his patients have told him they understood. The topics covered are those he was most often asked about by his patients and include how the heart works, what can go wrong, how it can be diagnosed and what can be done about it.

He has balanced the scientific presentation with reason and common sense, emphasizing not only the potential dangers of heart disease, but also the optimism that we can now share about the treatment of heart disease as a result of the remarkable progress and promise of medical science and technology.

Dr. Wise is certified by the American Board of Internal Medicine and by the Sub-Specialty Board of Cardiovascular Disease. He graduated from the University of Texas Southwestern Medical School, received his training in Internal Medicine at Parkland Hospital in Dallas and completed a Cardiology Fellowship at the Royal Postgraduate Medical School at Hammersmith Hospital in London.

He has been granted Fellowship in the American College of Cardiology, the American Heart Association Council on Clinical Cardiology and the American College of Physicians. For twenty-five years he practiced in Bangor, Maine where he was founder and managing partner of a fourteen-member cardiology group practice, Director of the Cardiac Catheterization Laboratory and Head of the Cardiology Section at Eastern Maine Medical Center, a 400-bed regional medical center.

Dr. Wise has made numerous contributions to the cardiology literature including twenty-eight scientific articles and a book chapter on congenital heart disease. Currently he lives with his wife in Santa Fe where he is an associate with Southwest Cardiology Associates.

INDEX

~